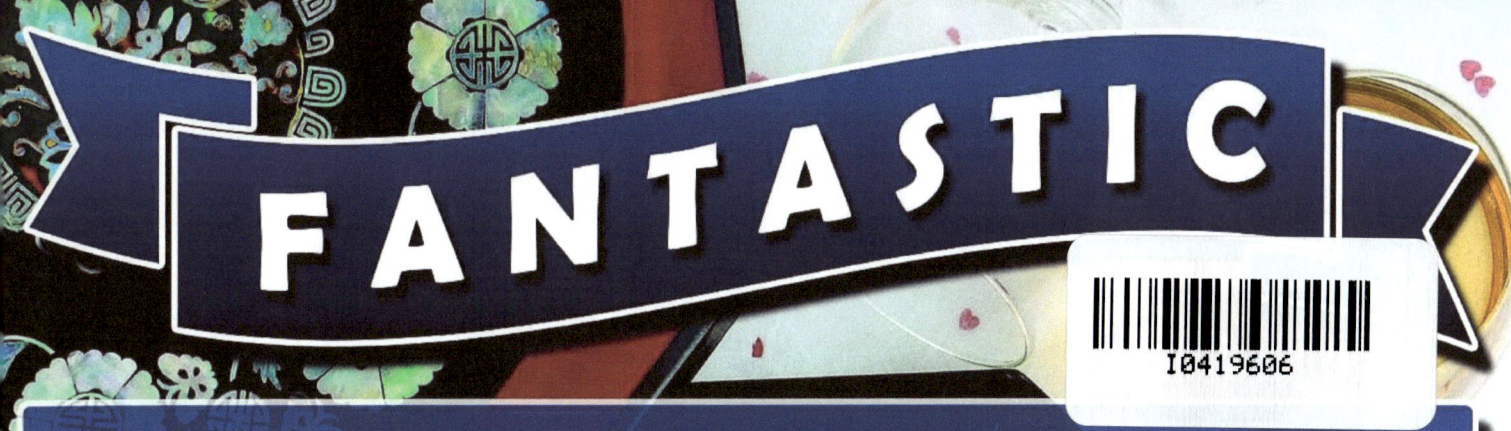

FANTASTIC

I0419606

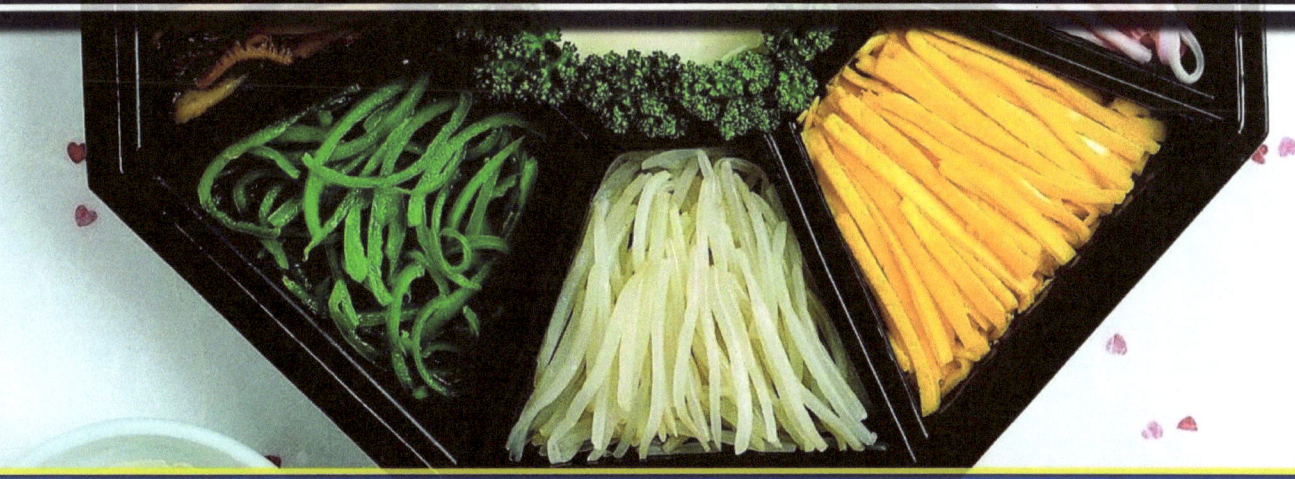

FOOD & DESSERTS

40 FULL COLOR IMAGES

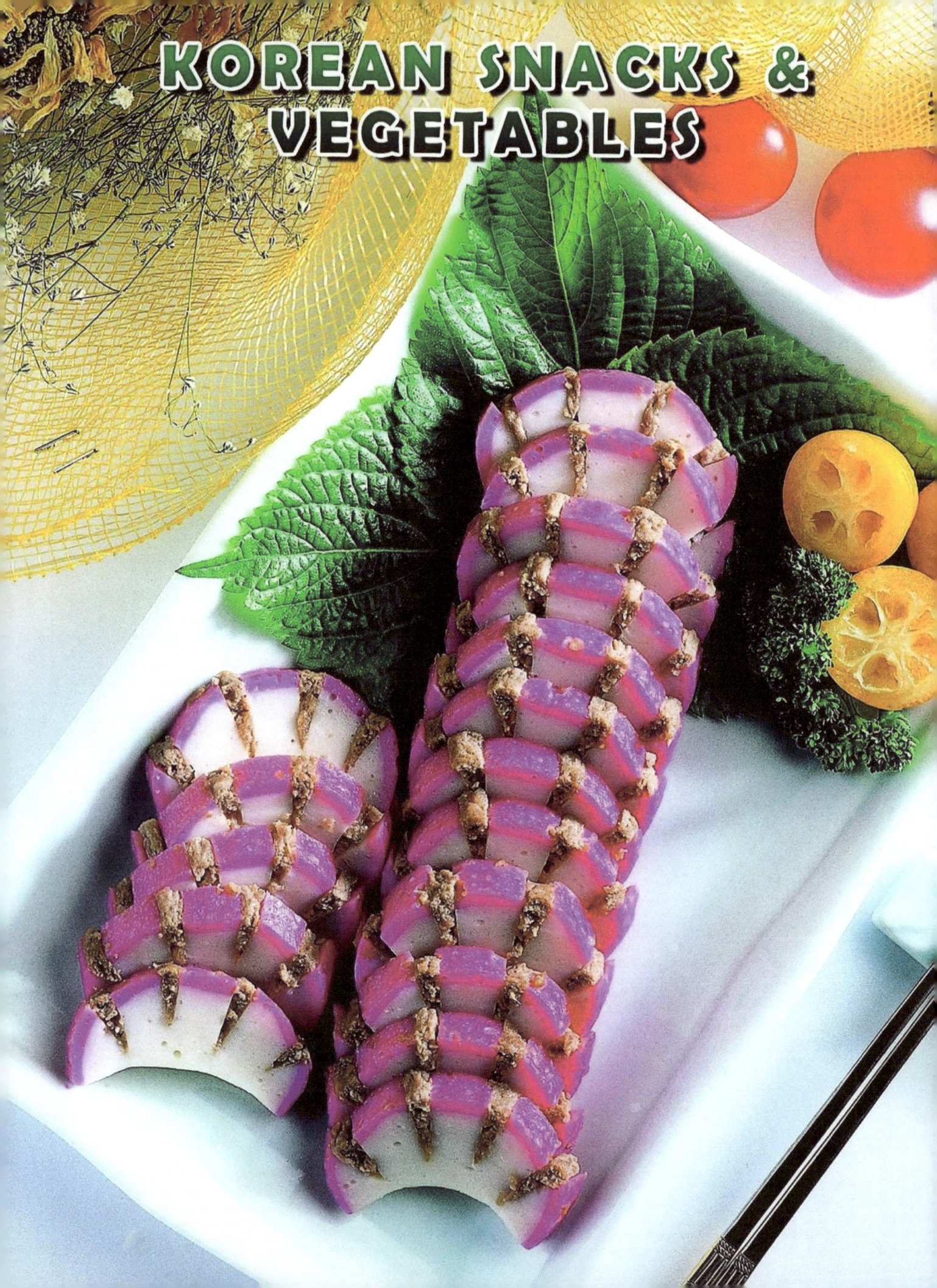

KOREAN SNACKS & VEGETABLES

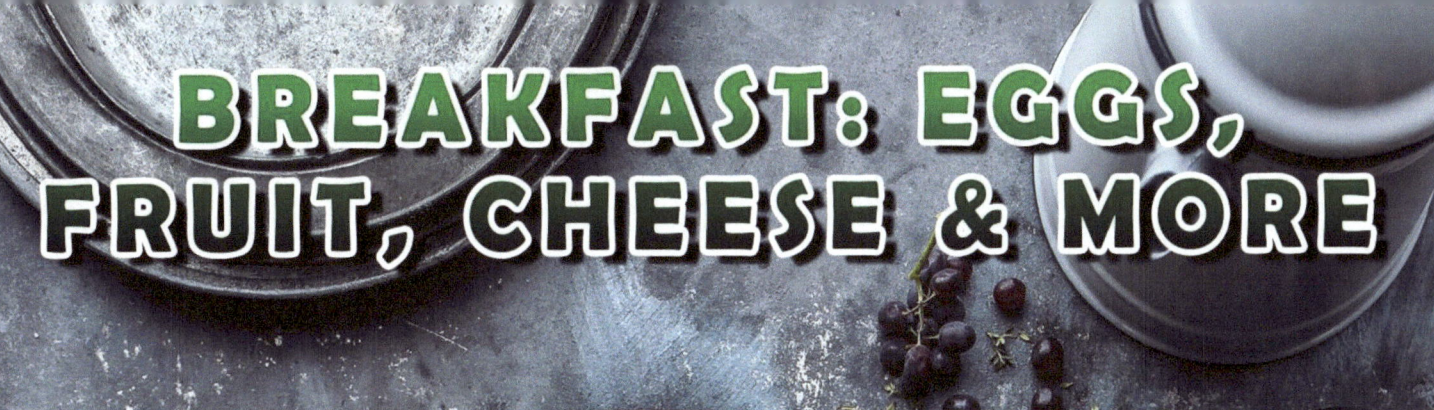

BREAKFAST: EGGS, FRUIT, CHEESE & MORE

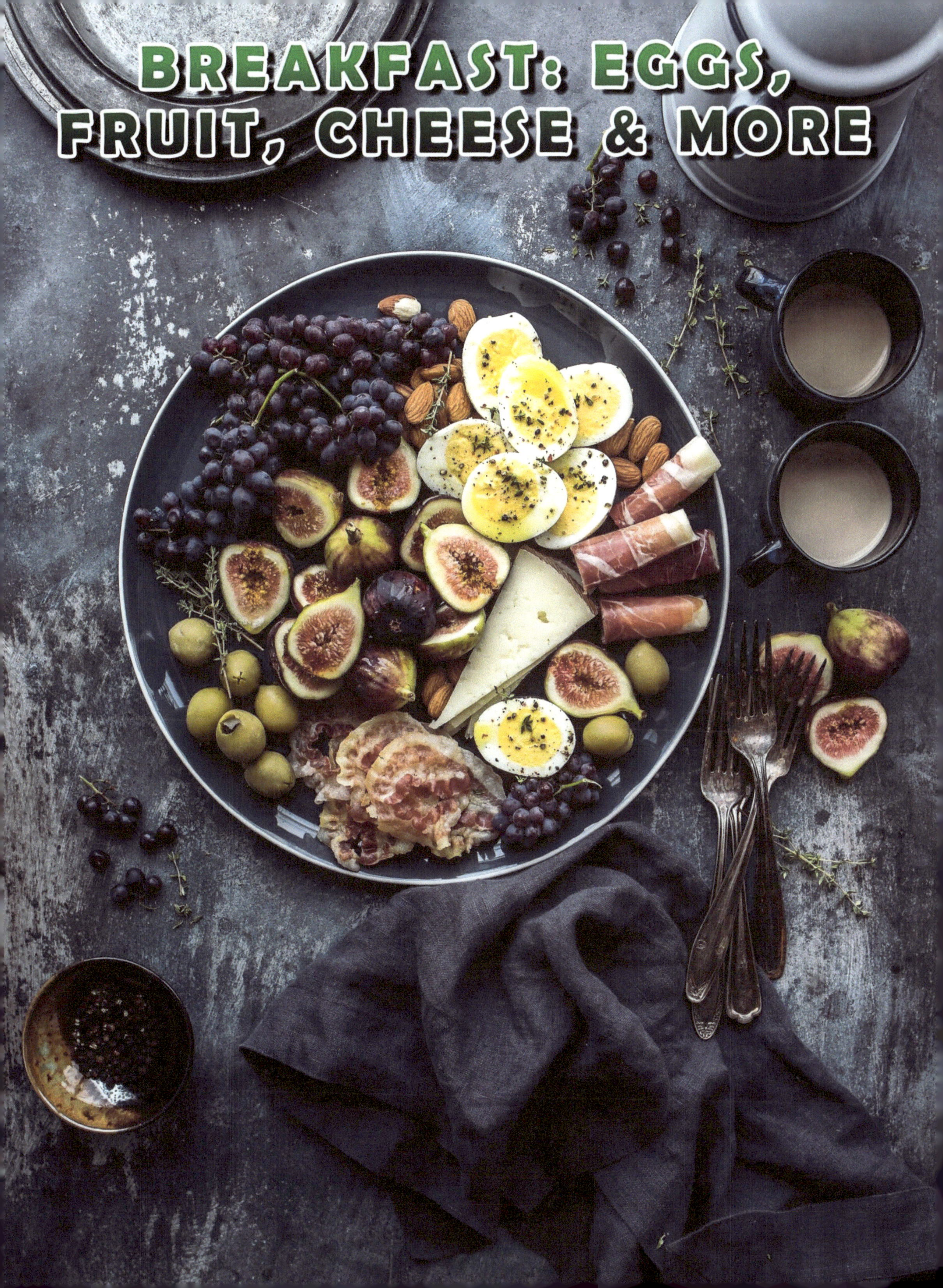

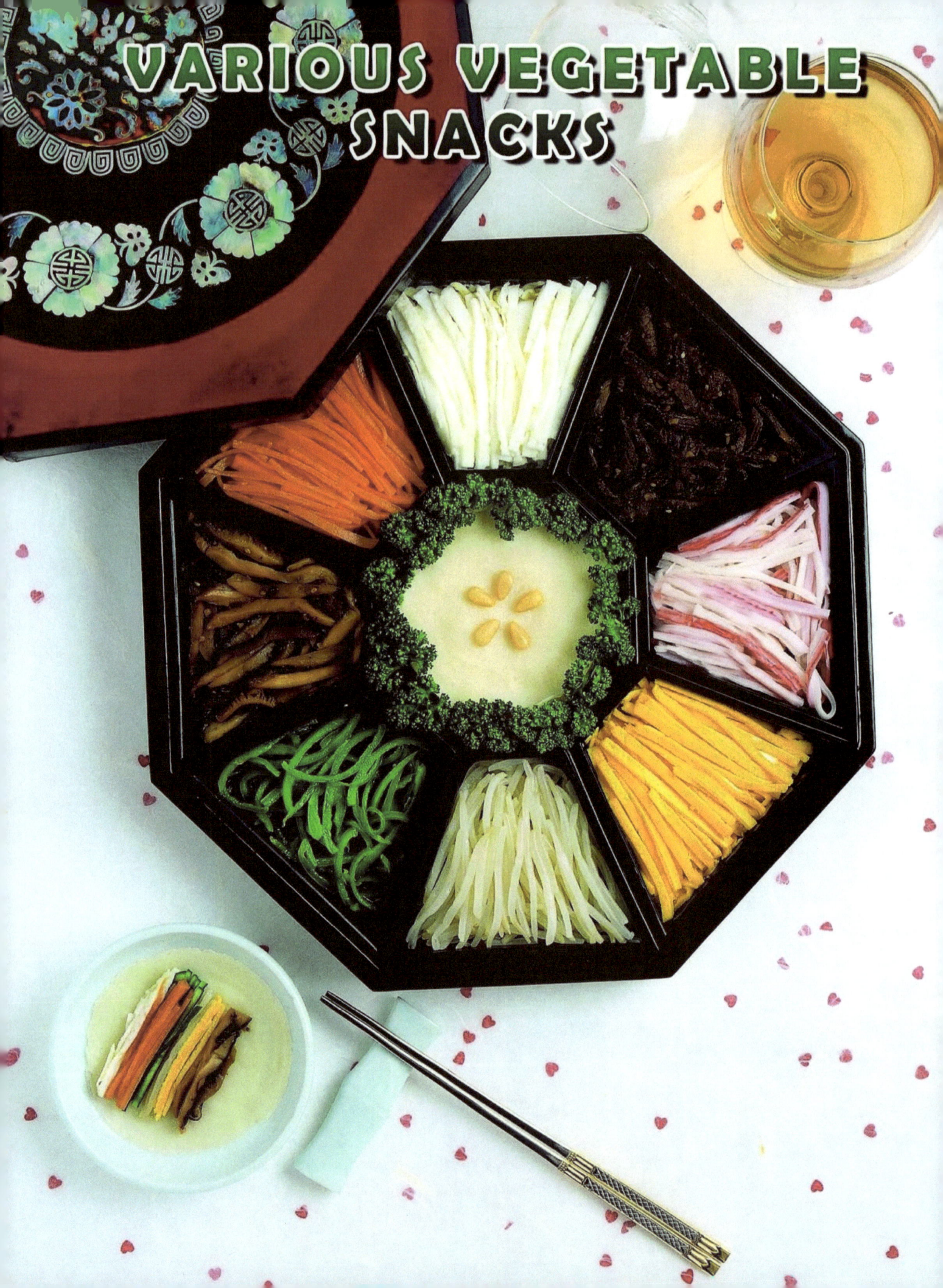

VARIOUS VEGETABLE SNACKS

VARIOUS HERBS

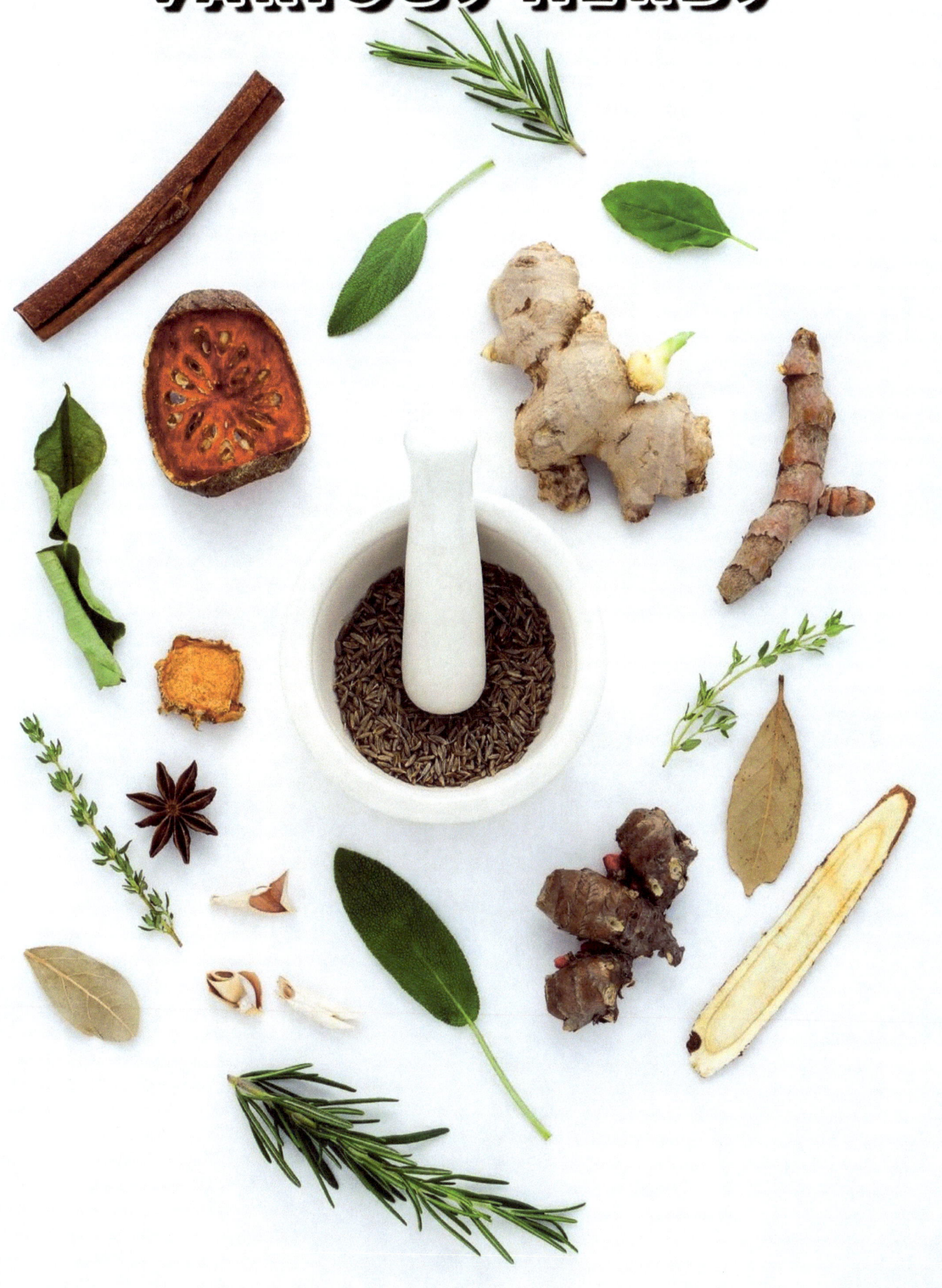

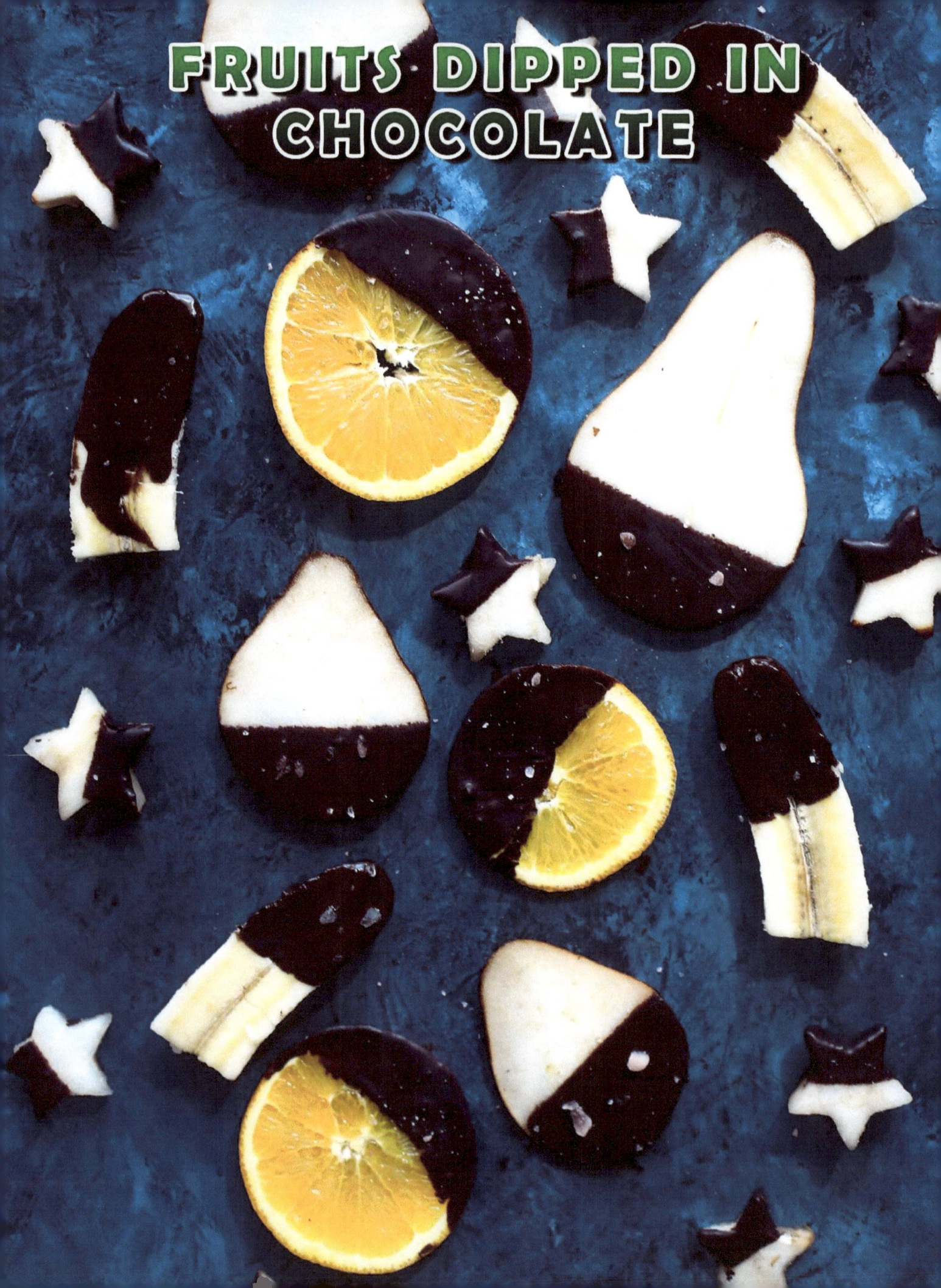

FRUITS DIPPED IN CHOCOLATE

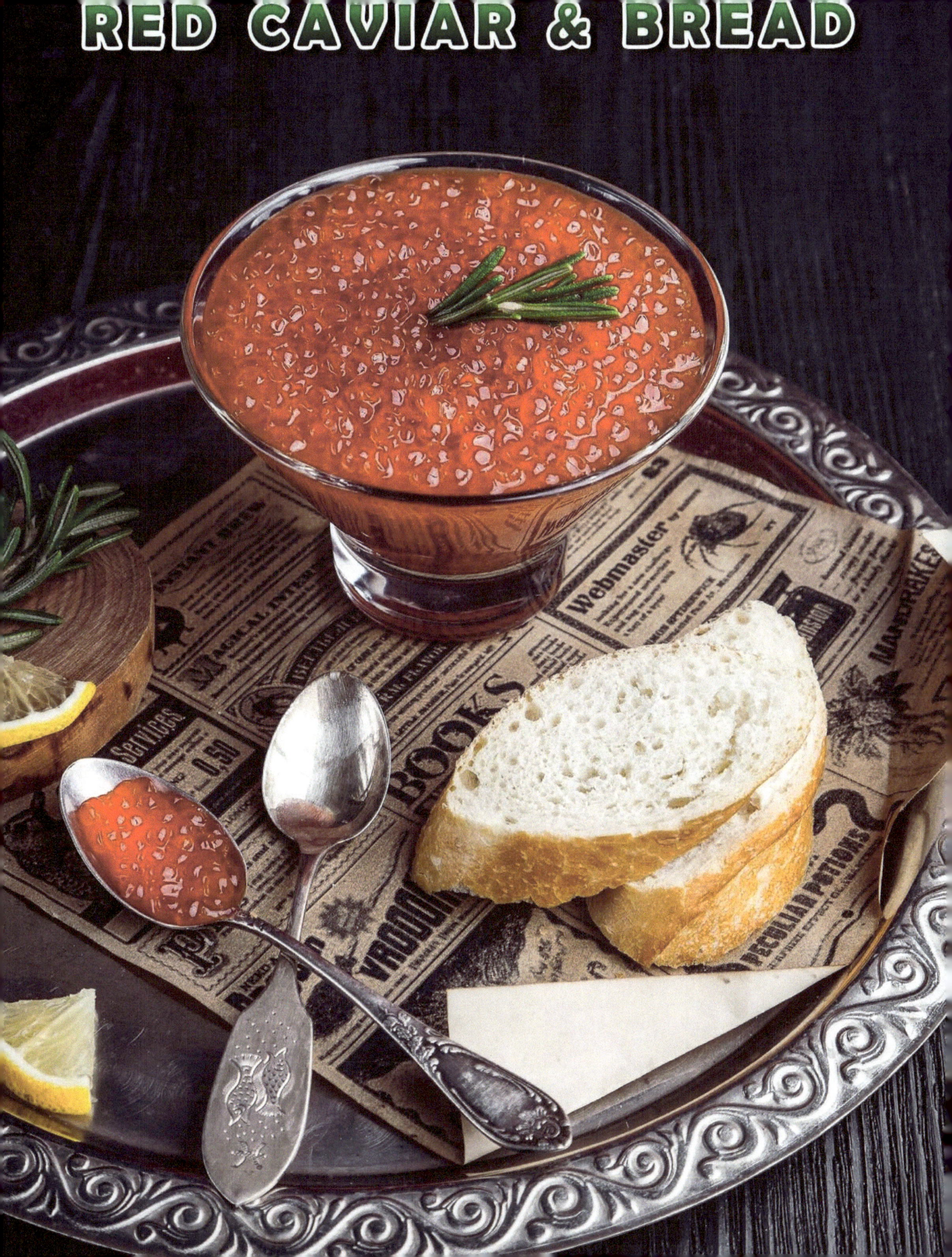

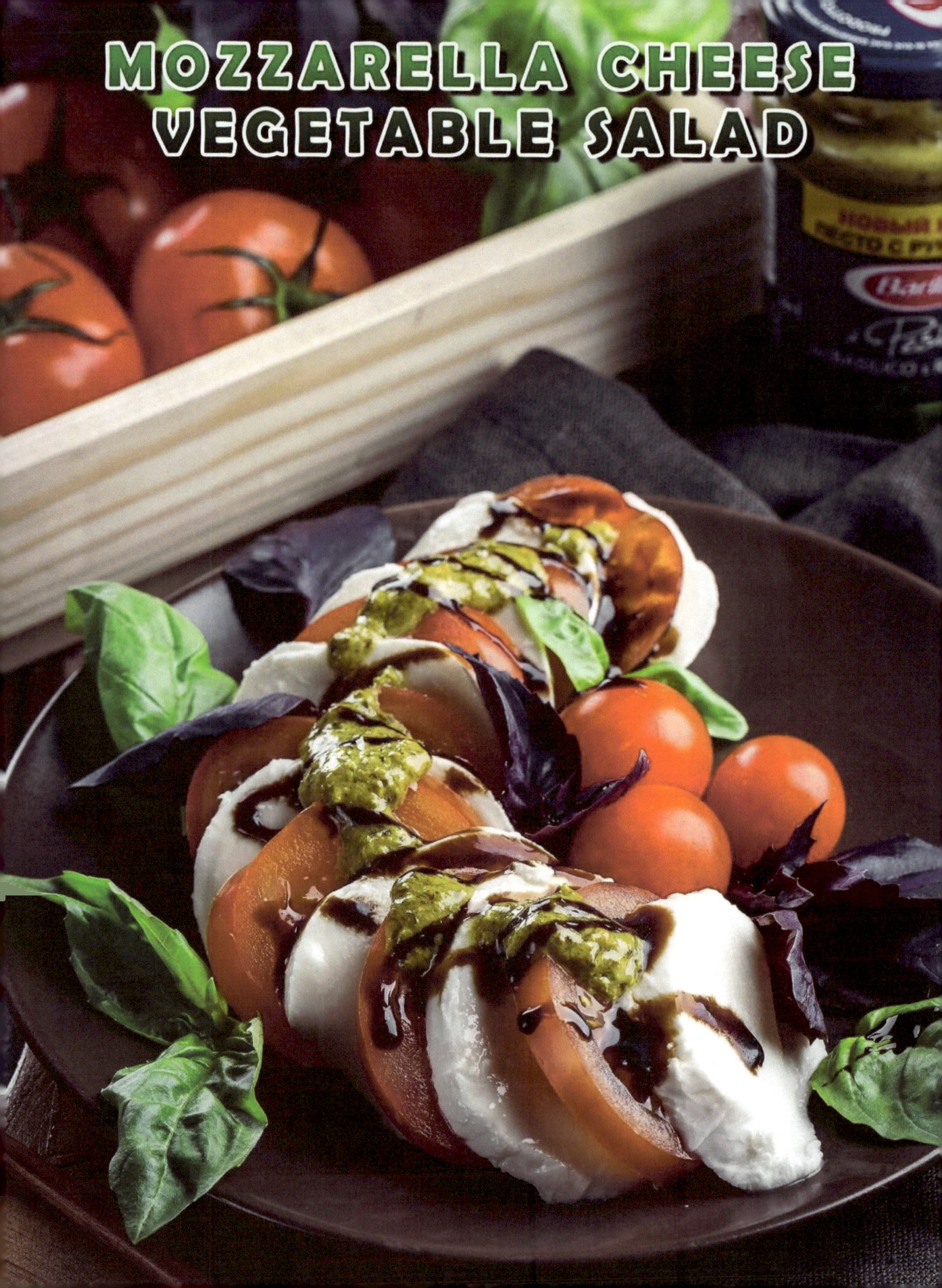

MOZZARELLA CHEESE VEGETABLE SALAD

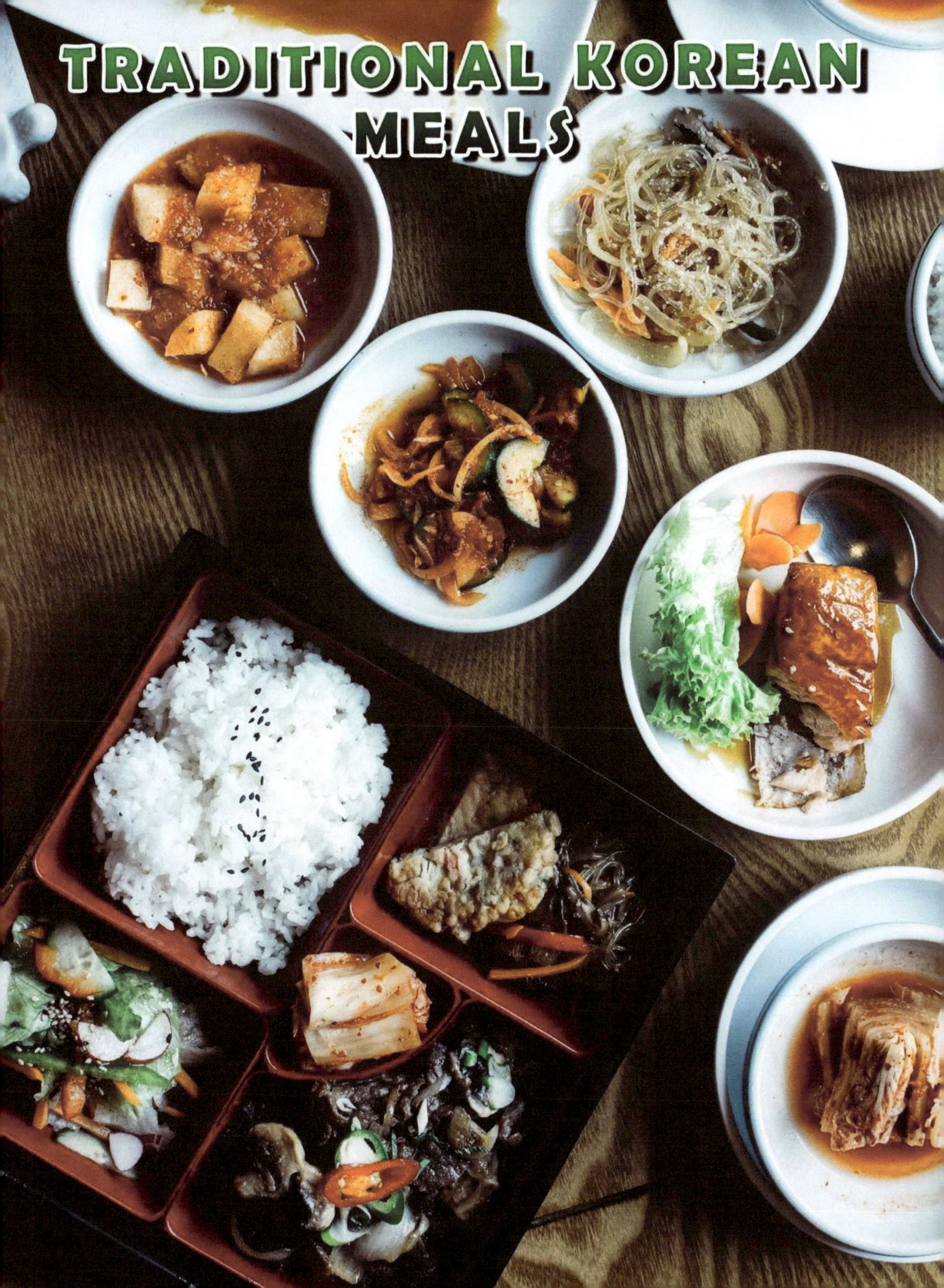

TRADITIONAL KOREAN MEALS

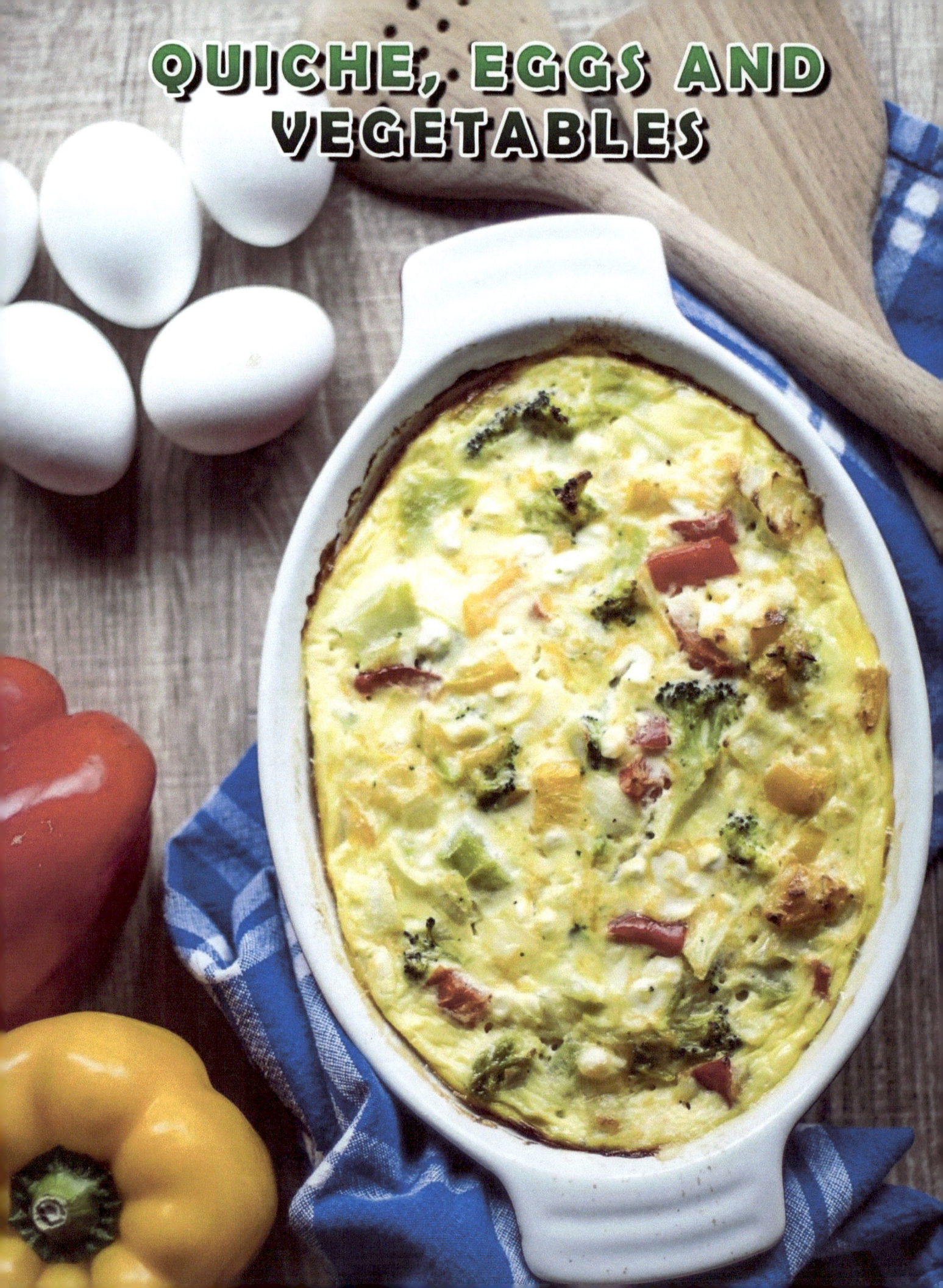

QUICHE, EGGS AND VEGETABLES

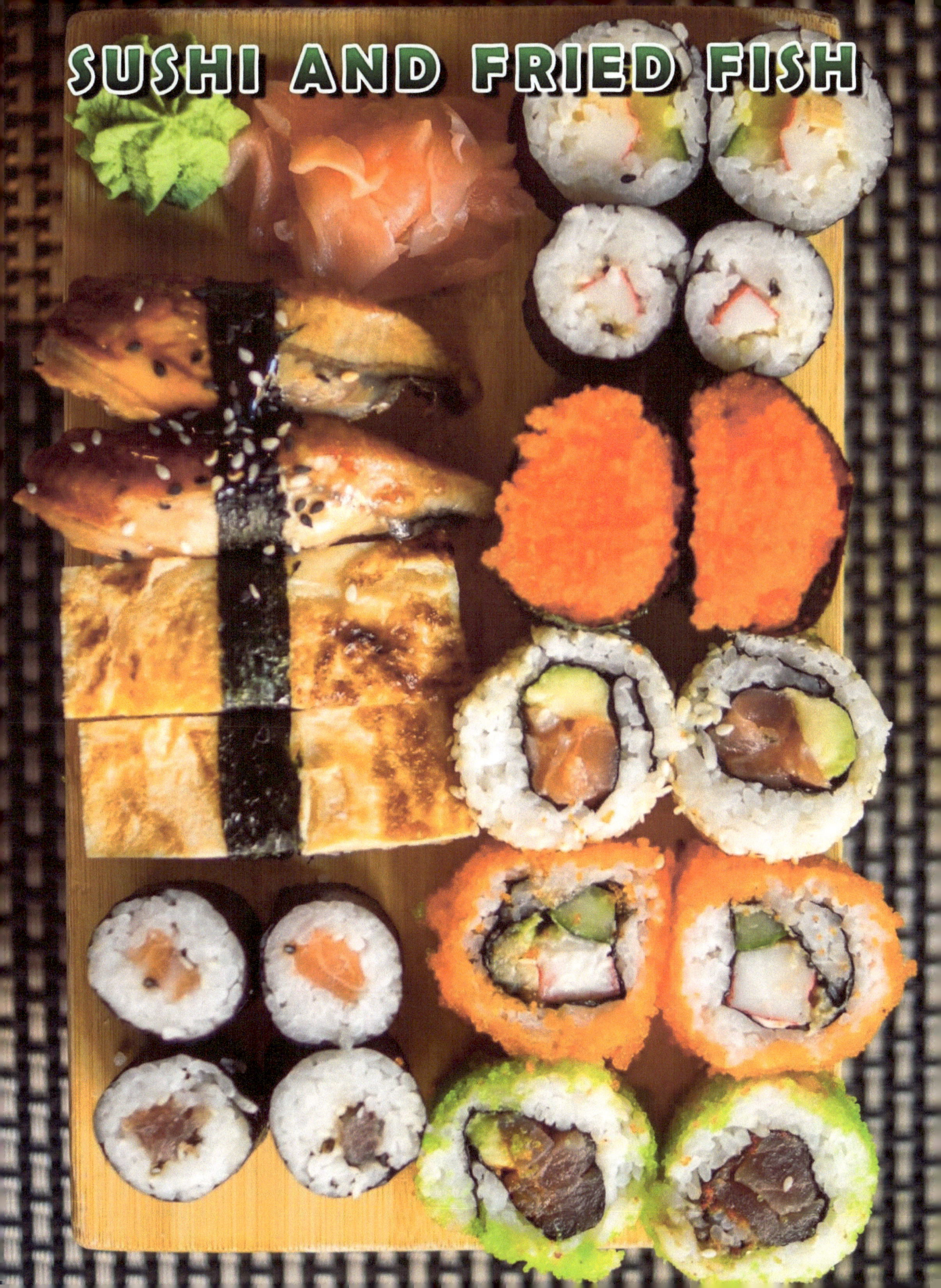

SUSHI AND FRIED FISH

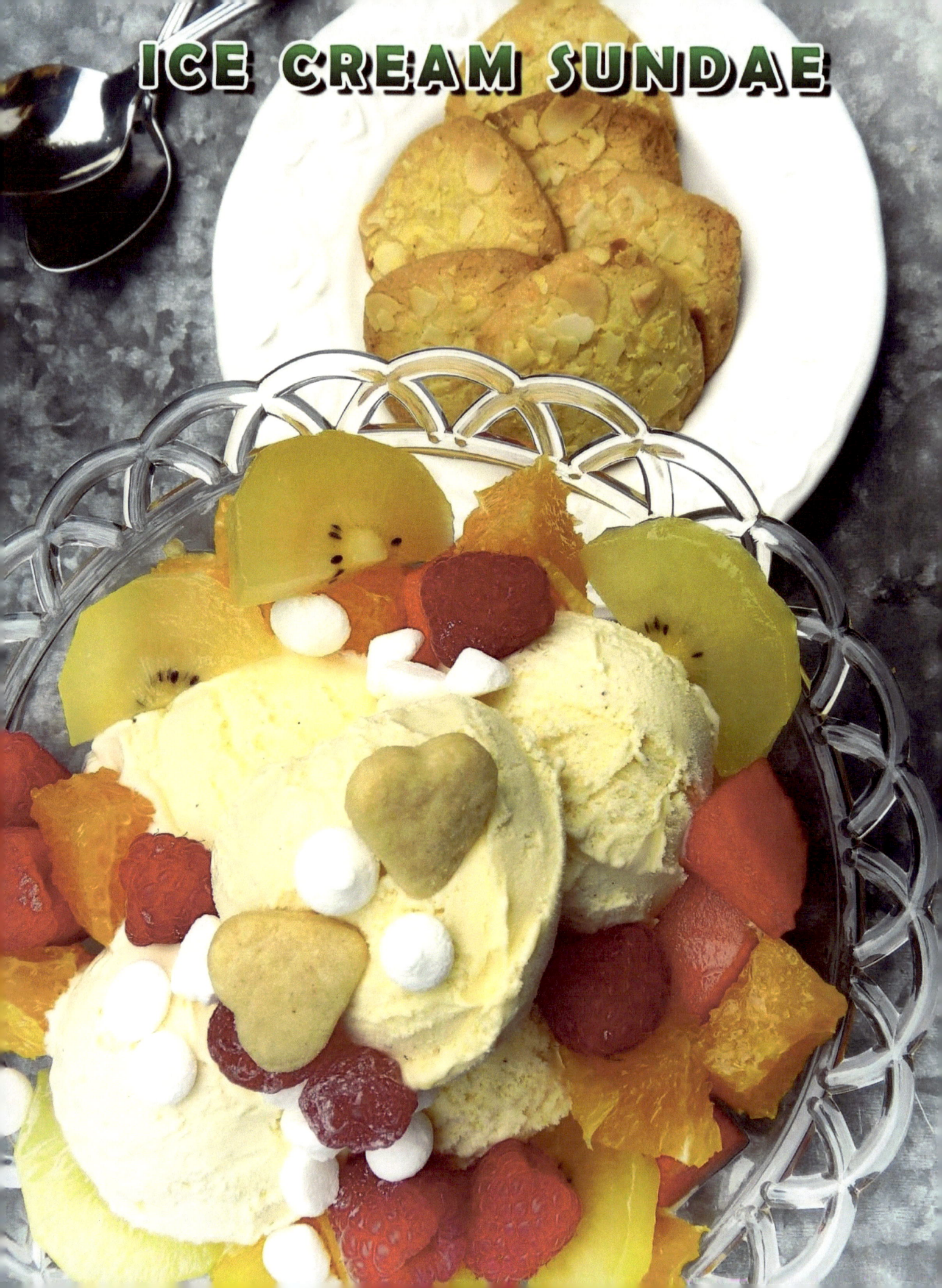

ICE CREAM SUNDAE

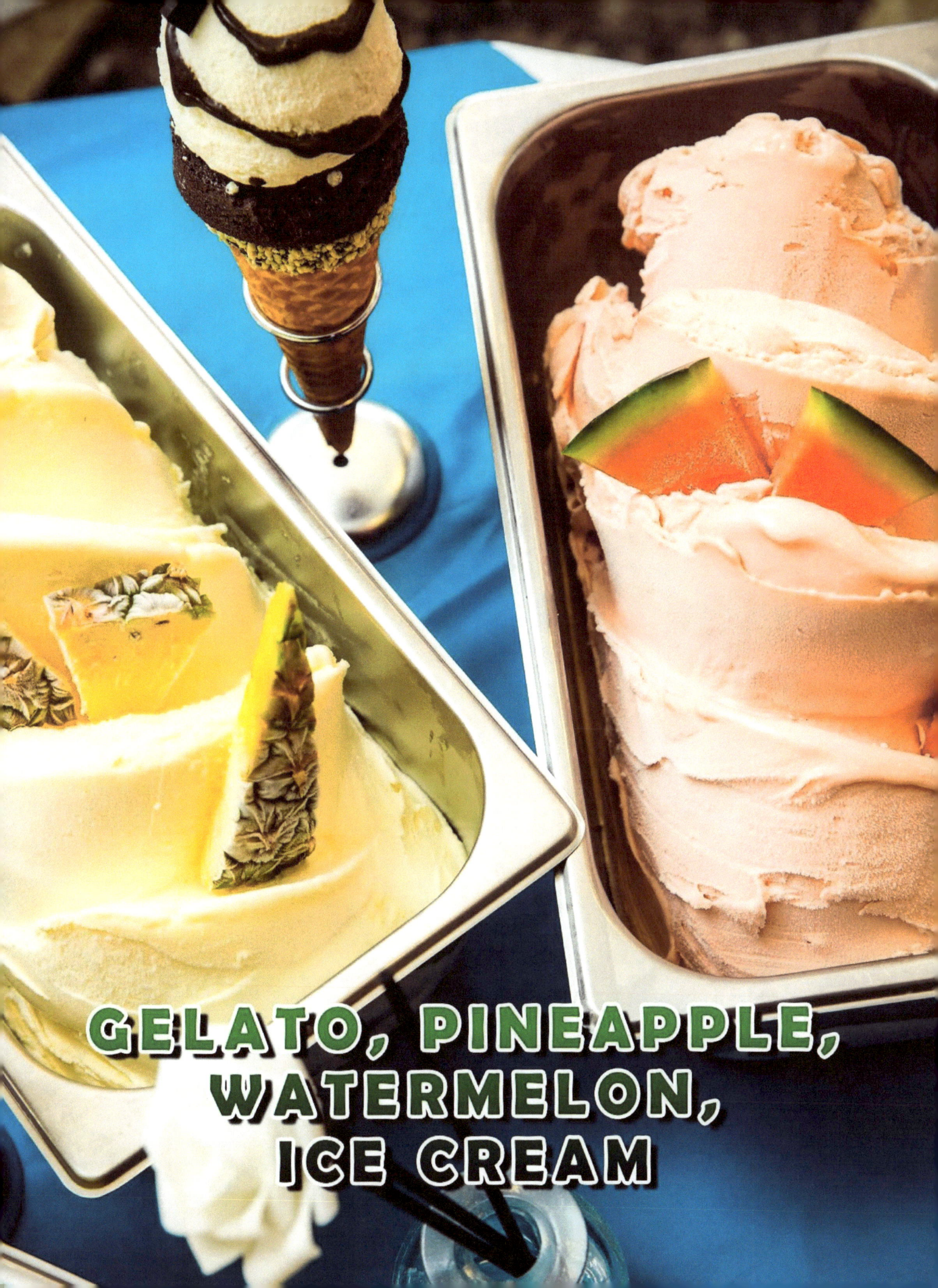

GELATO, PINEAPPLE, WATERMELON, ICE CREAM

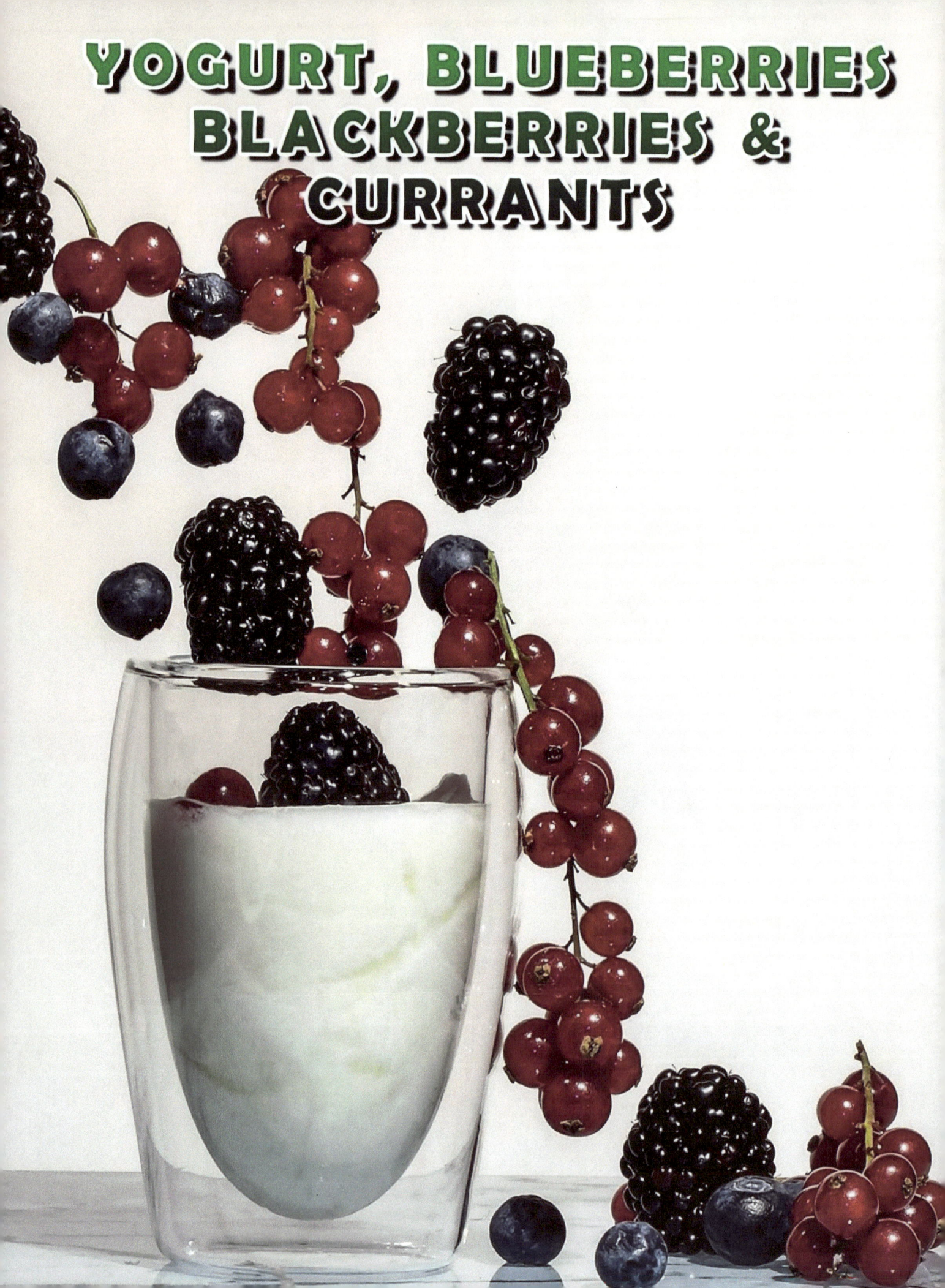

YOGURT, BLUEBERRIES BLACKBERRIES & CURRANTS

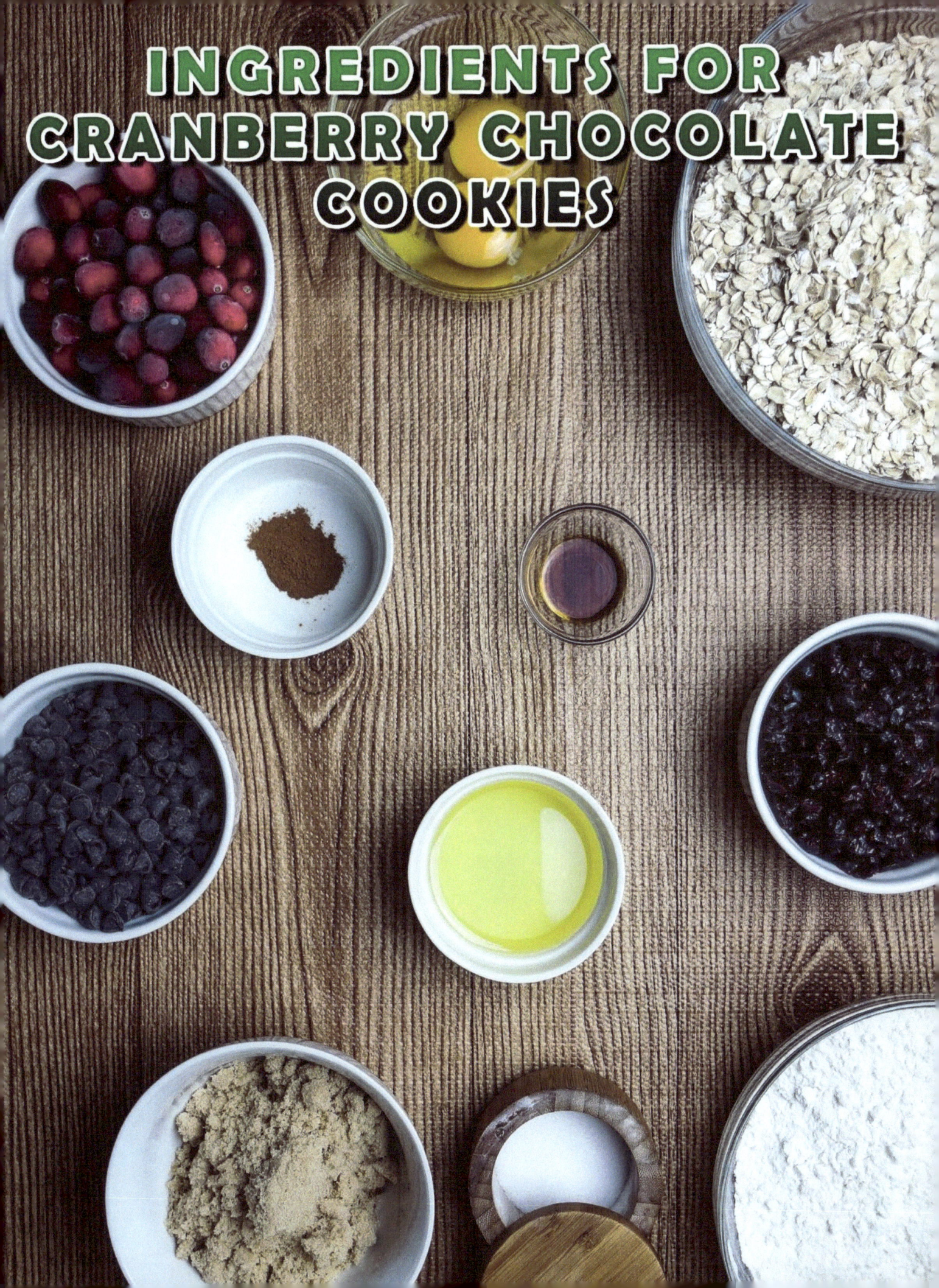

INGREDIENTS FOR CRANBERRY CHOCOLATE COOKIES

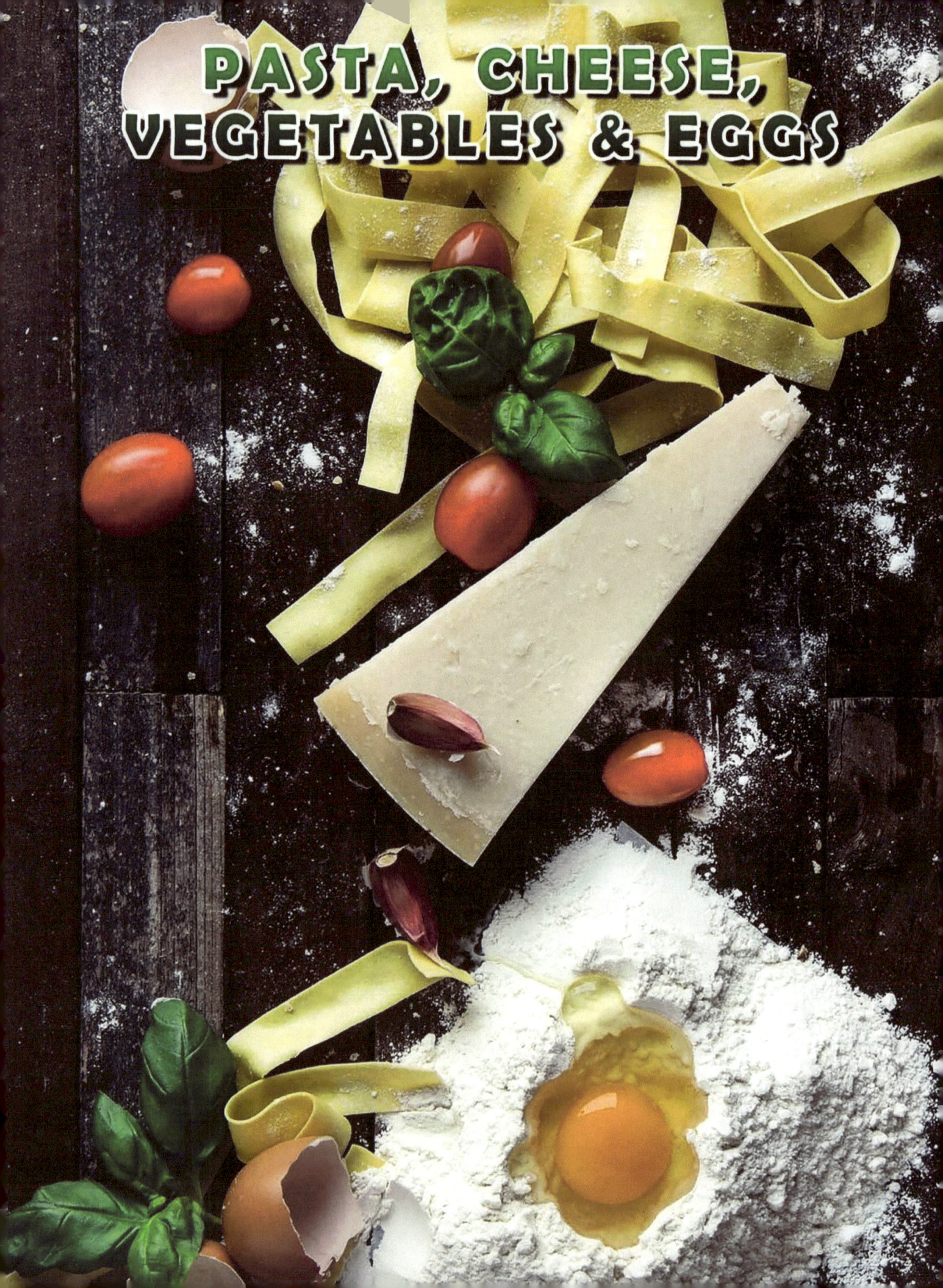

PASTA, CHEESE, VEGETABLES & EGGS

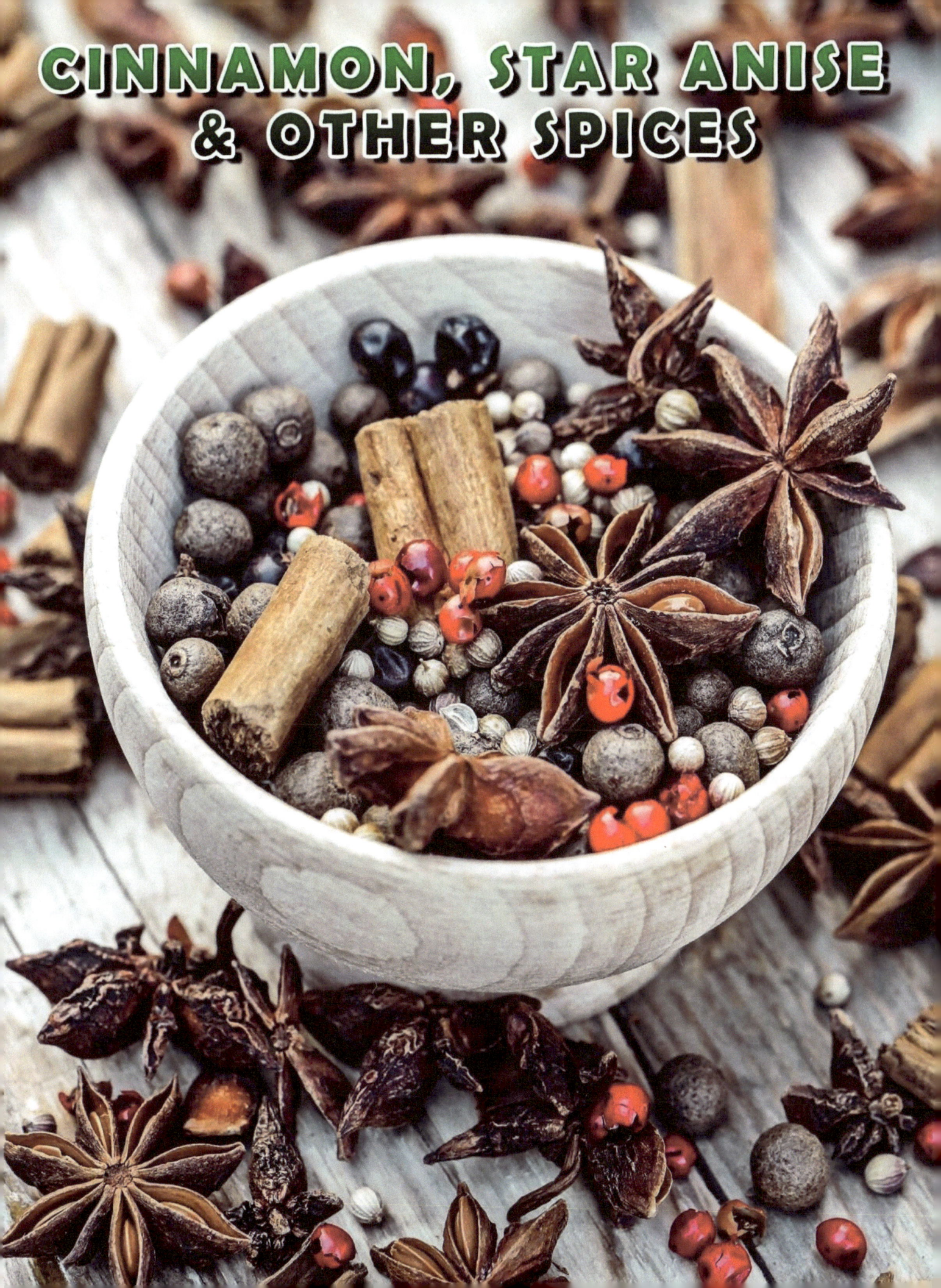

CINNAMON, STAR ANISE & OTHER SPICES

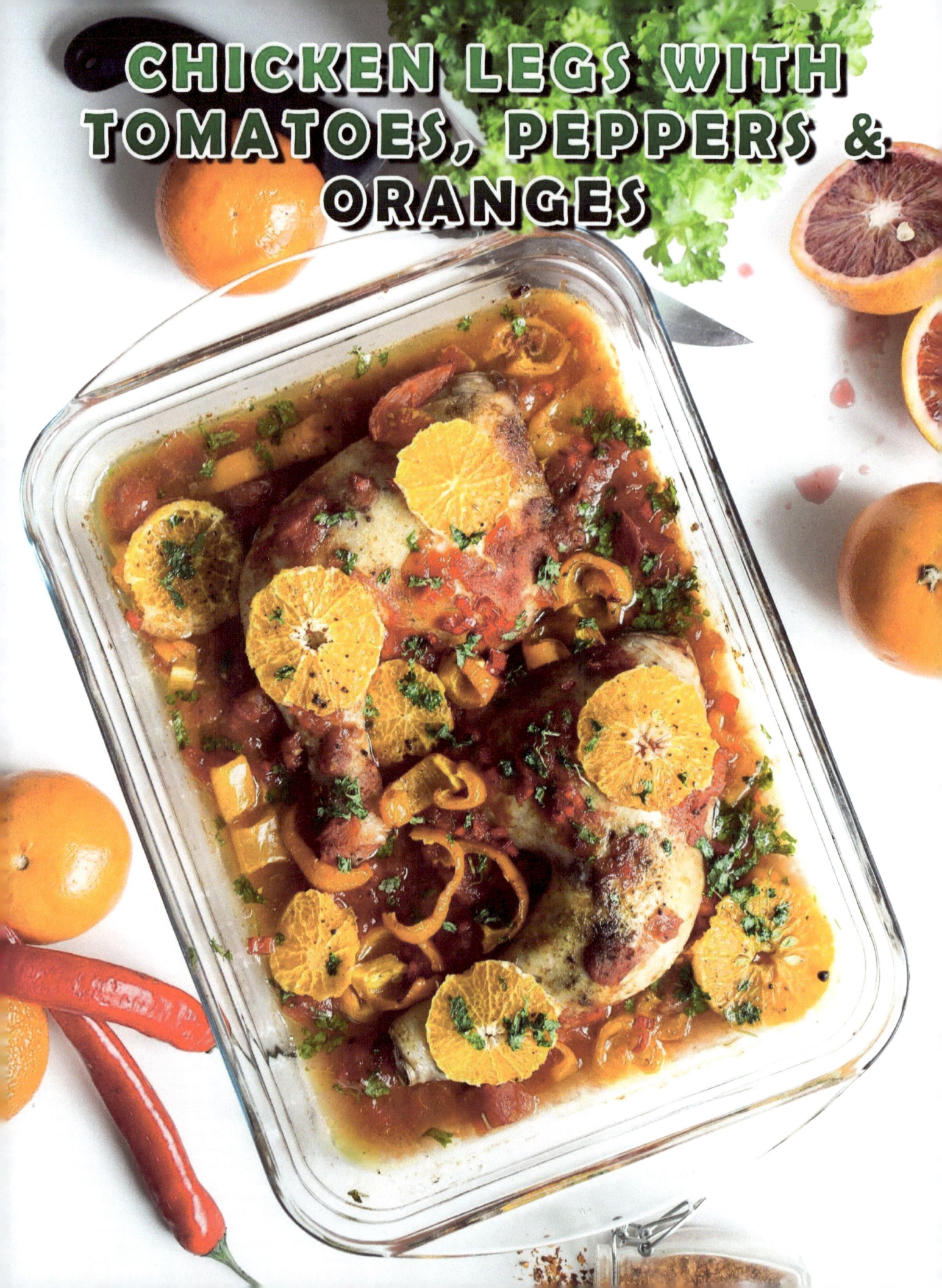

CHICKEN LEGS WITH TOMATOES, PEPPERS & ORANGES

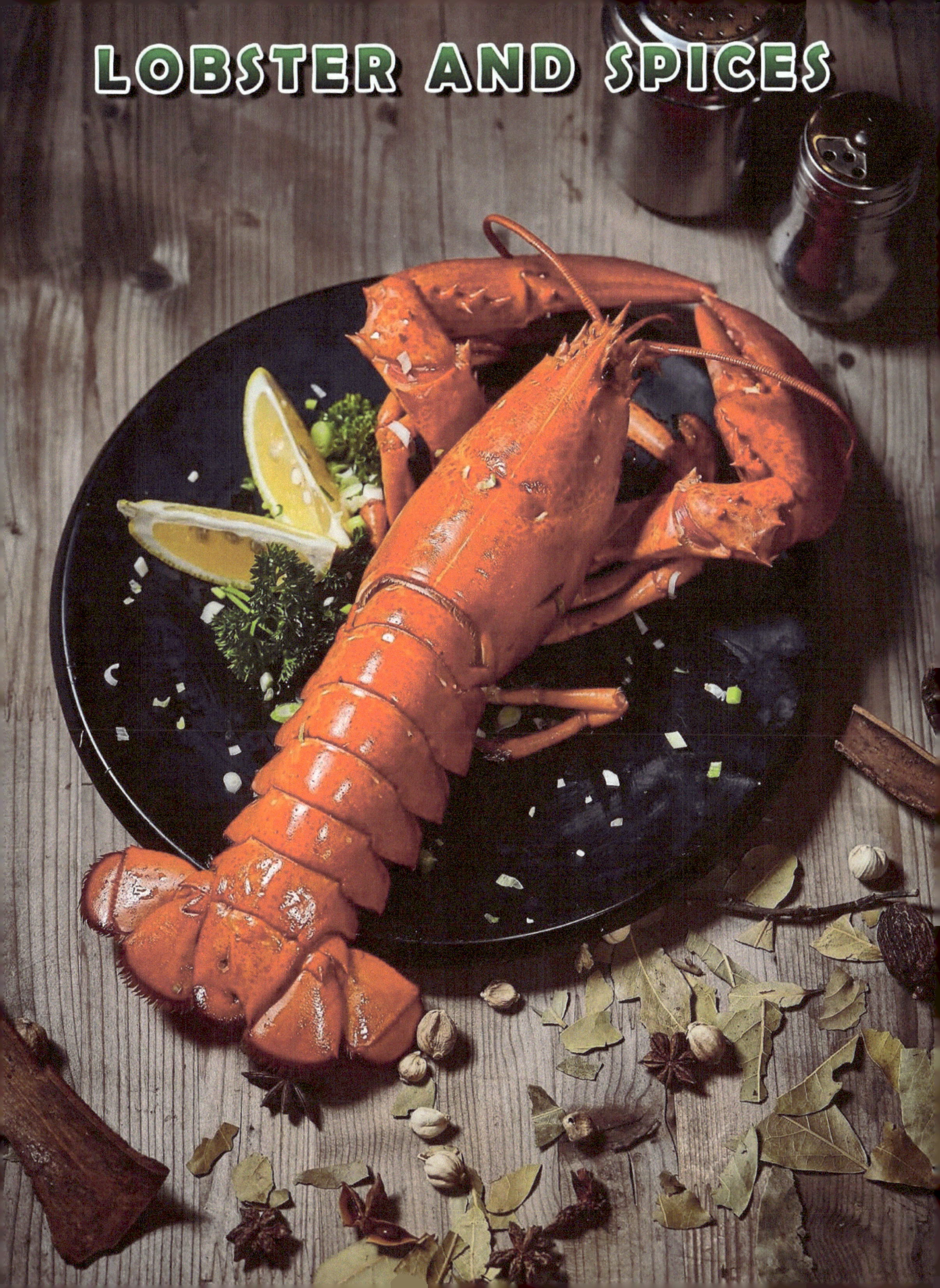

LOBSTER AND SPICES

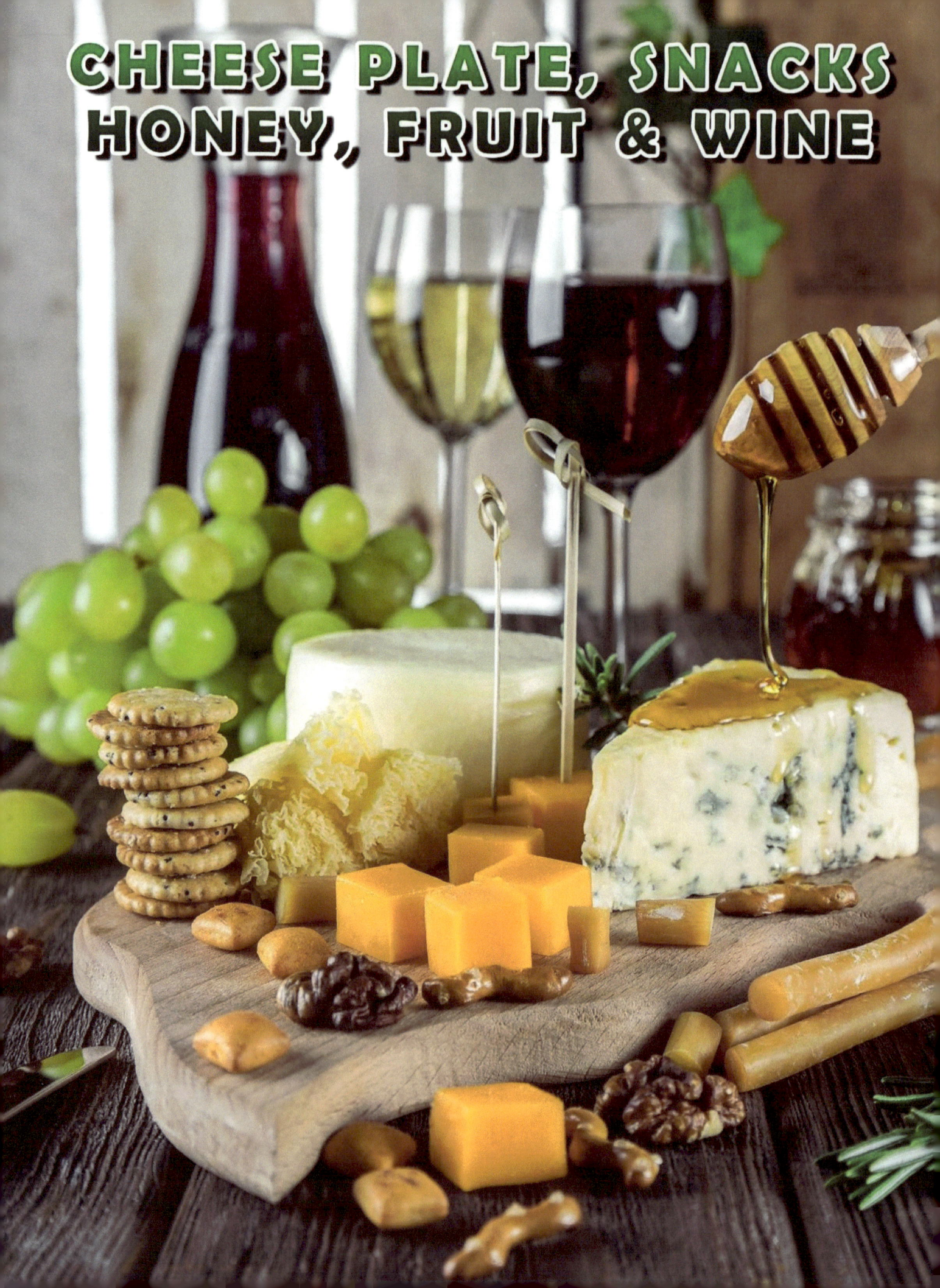

CHEESE PLATE, SNACKS HONEY, FRUIT & WINE

CREPE (A TYPE OF VERY THIN PANCAKE)

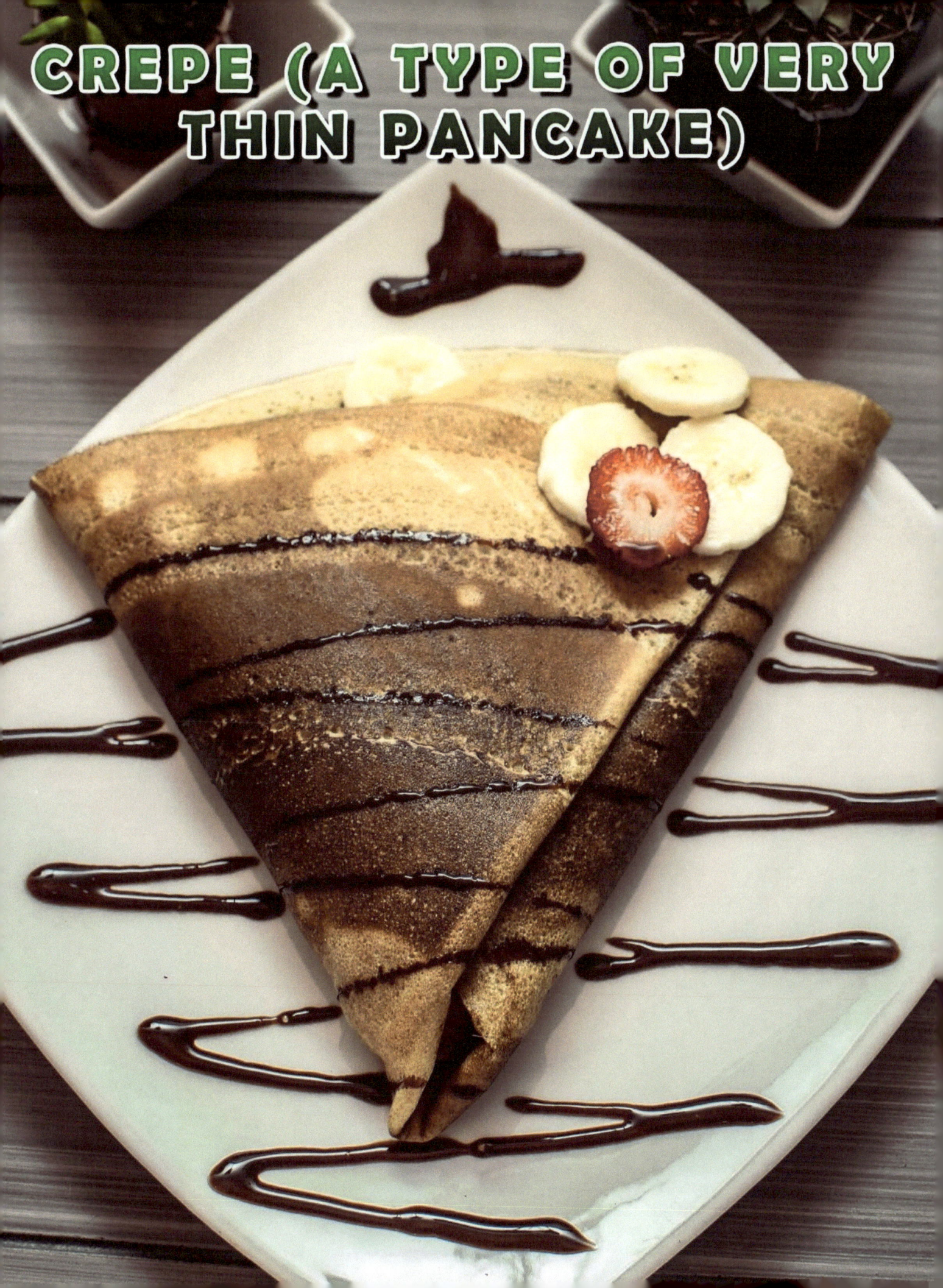

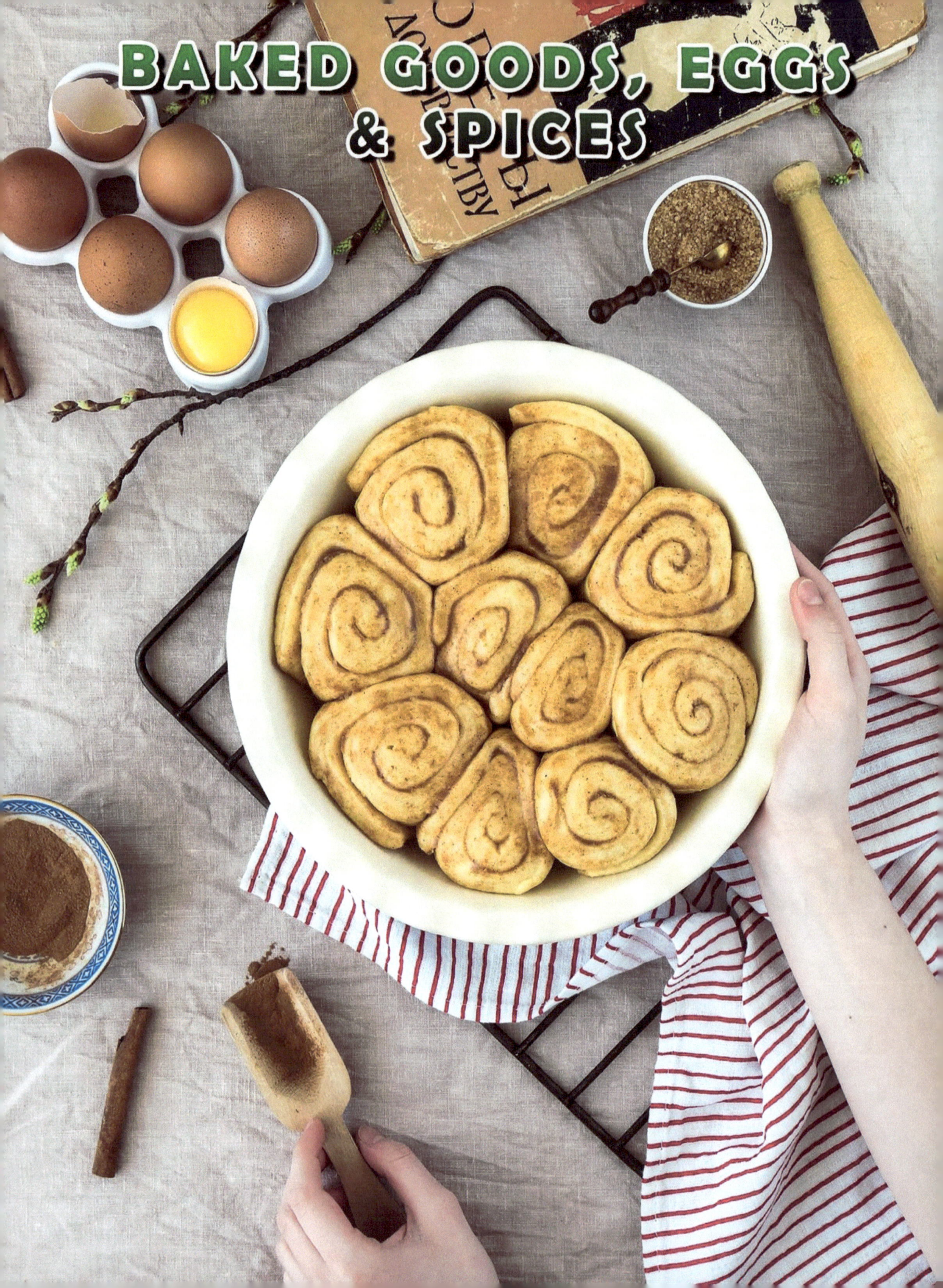

BAKED GOODS, EGGS & SPICES

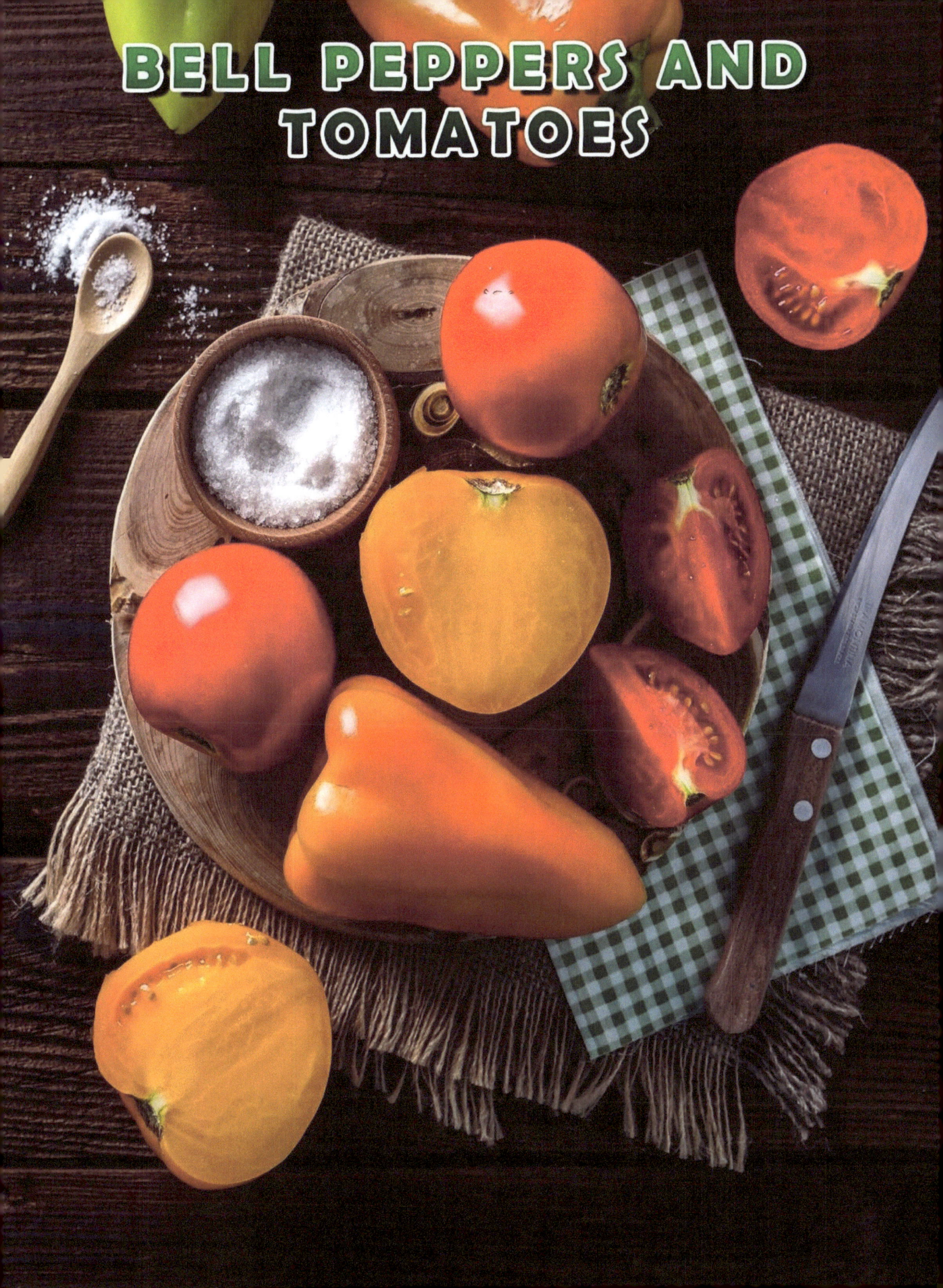

BELL PEPPERS AND TOMATOES

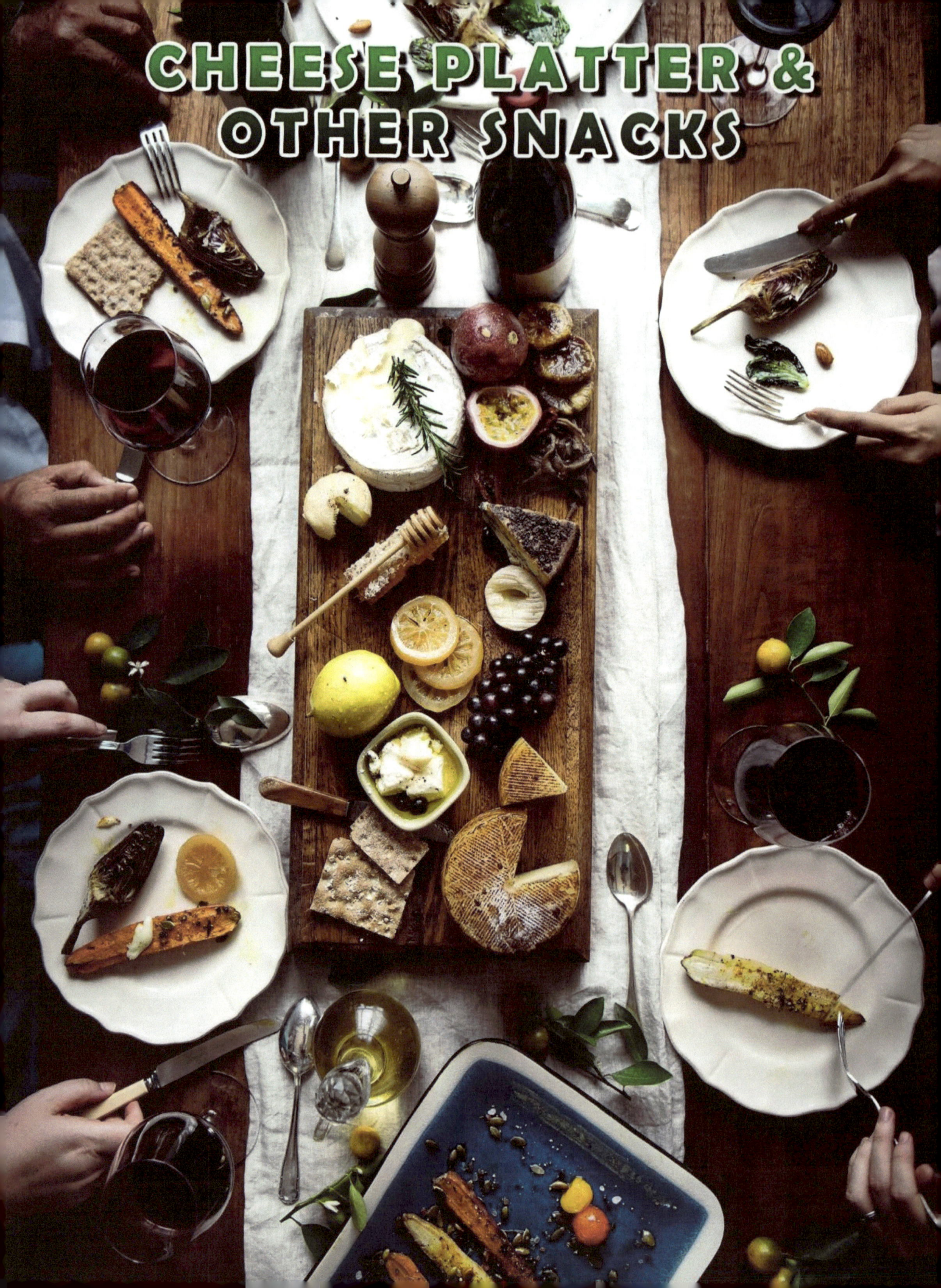

CHEESE PLATTER & OTHER SNACKS

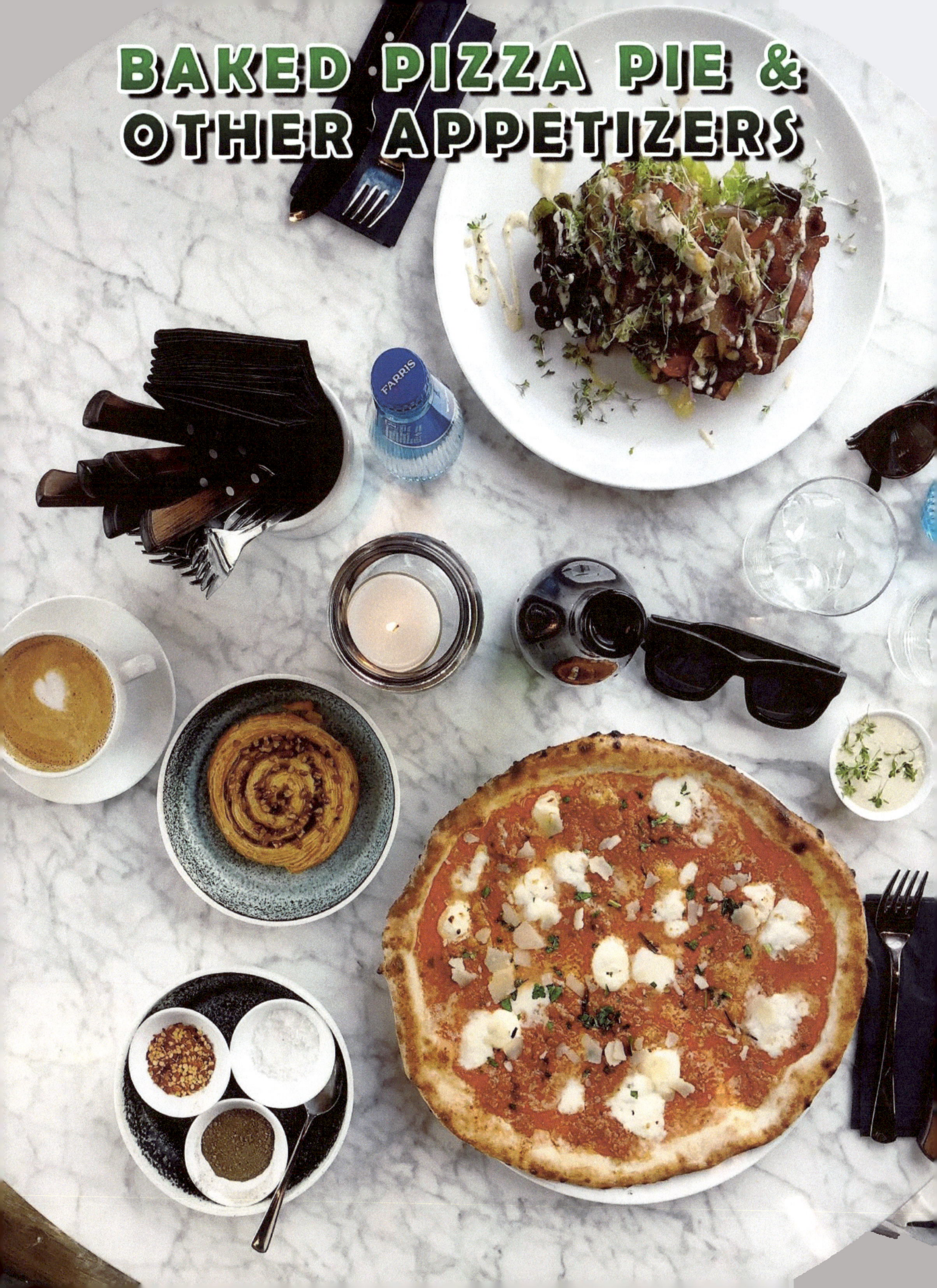

BAKED PIZZA PIE & OTHER APPETIZERS

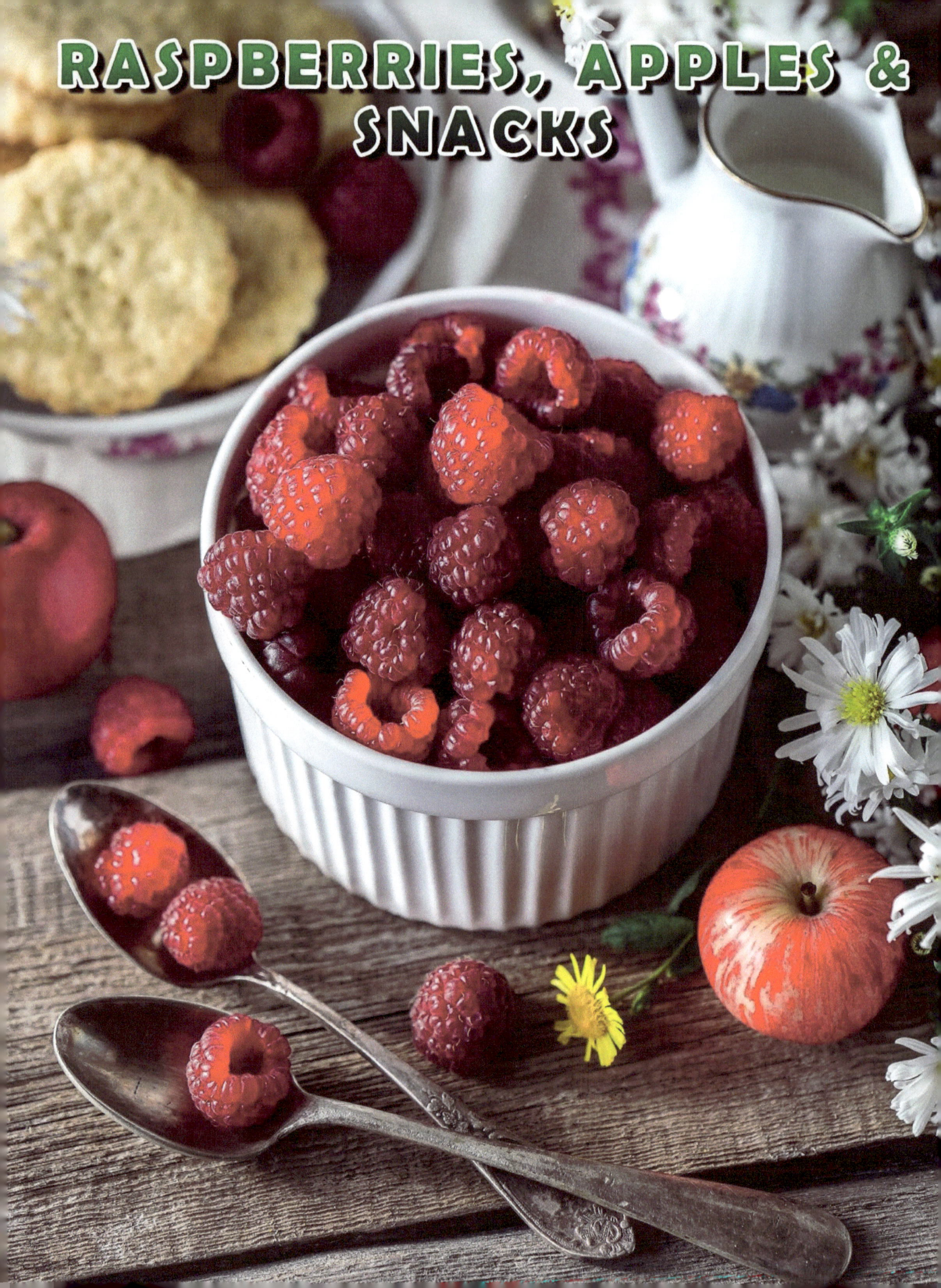

RASPBERRIES, APPLES & SNACKS

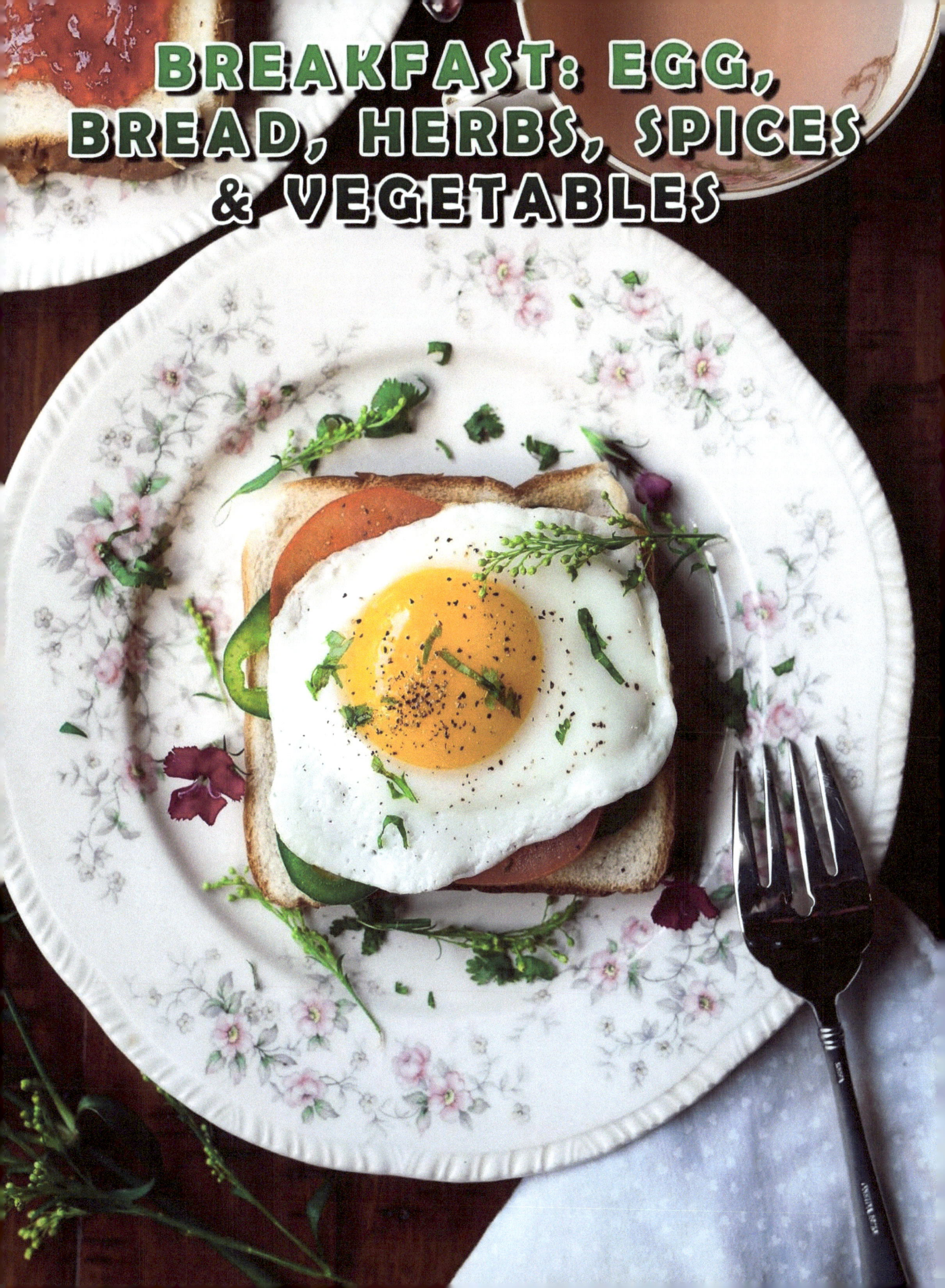

BREAKFAST: EGG, BREAD, HERBS, SPICES & VEGETABLES

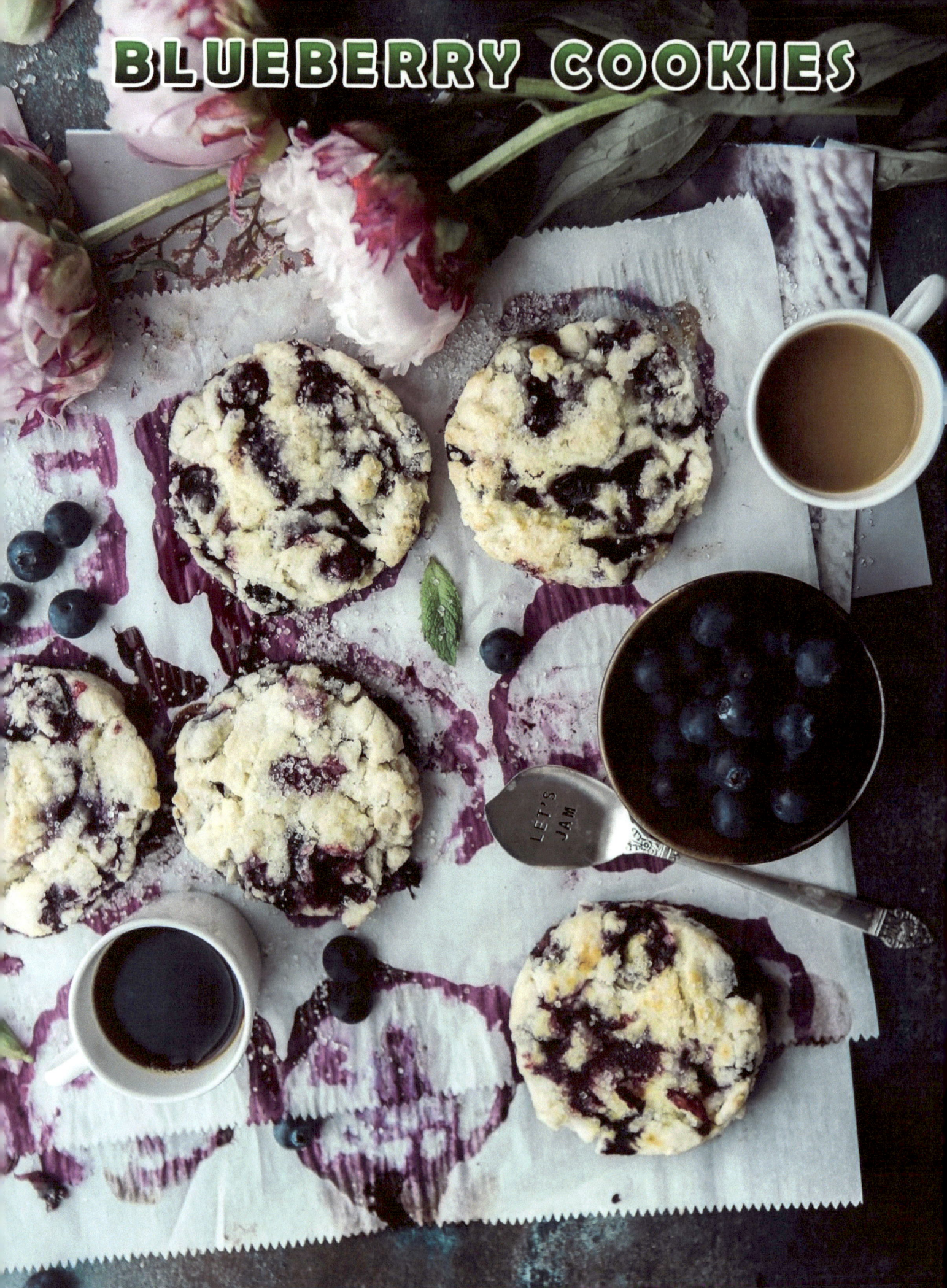

BLUEBERRY COOKIES

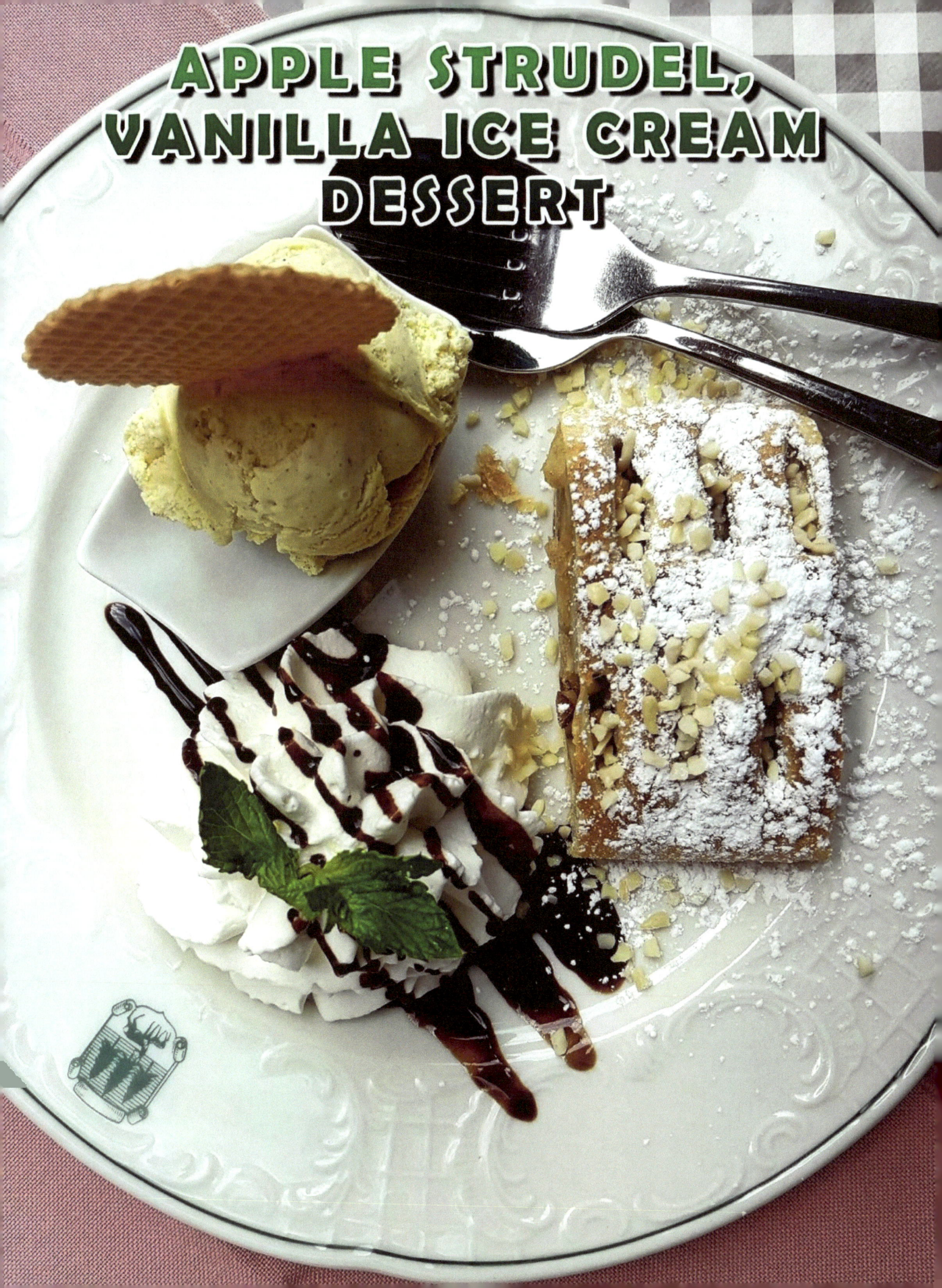

APPLE STRUDEL, VANILLA ICE CREAM DESSERT

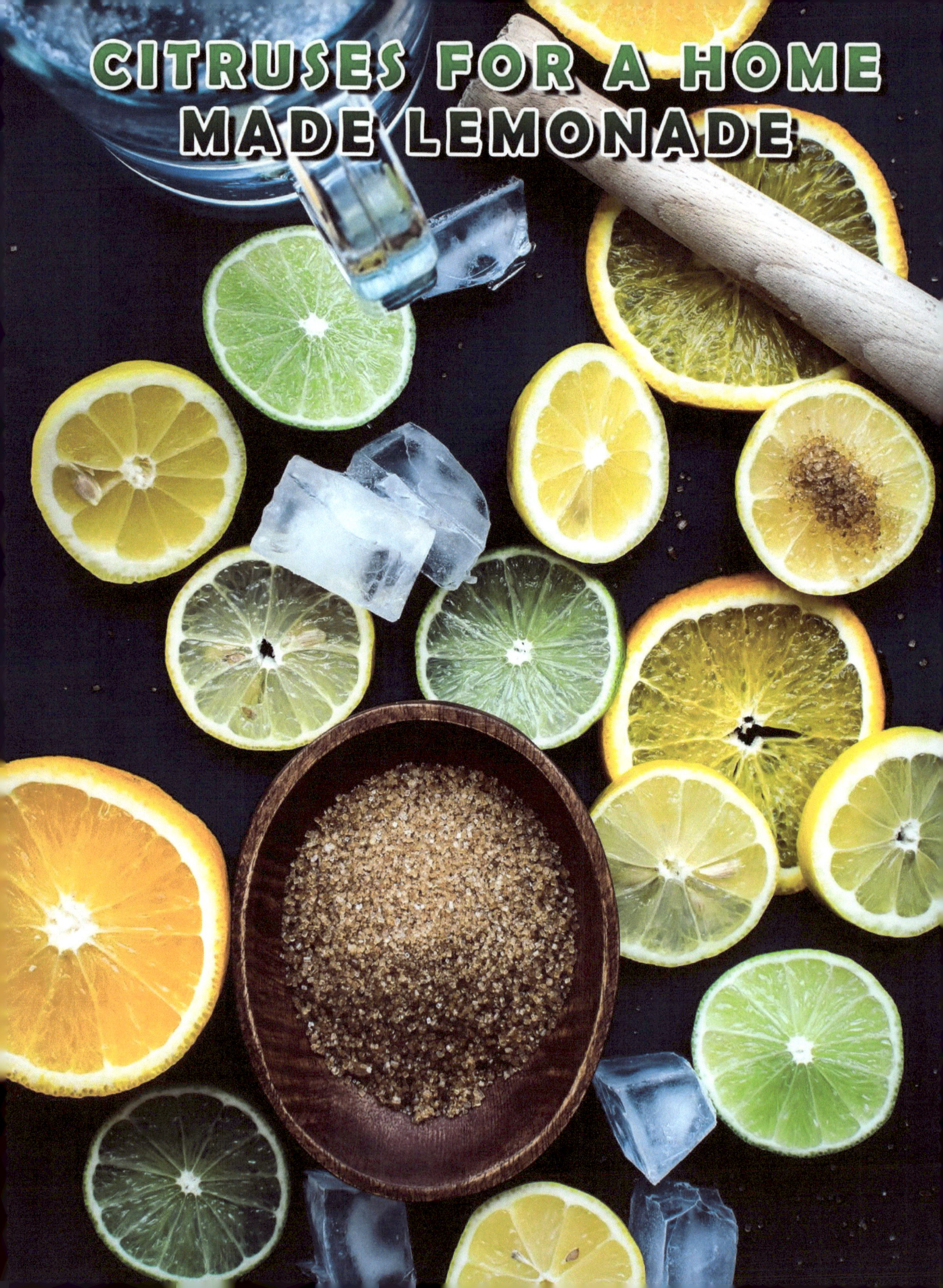

CITRUSES FOR A HOME MADE LEMONADE

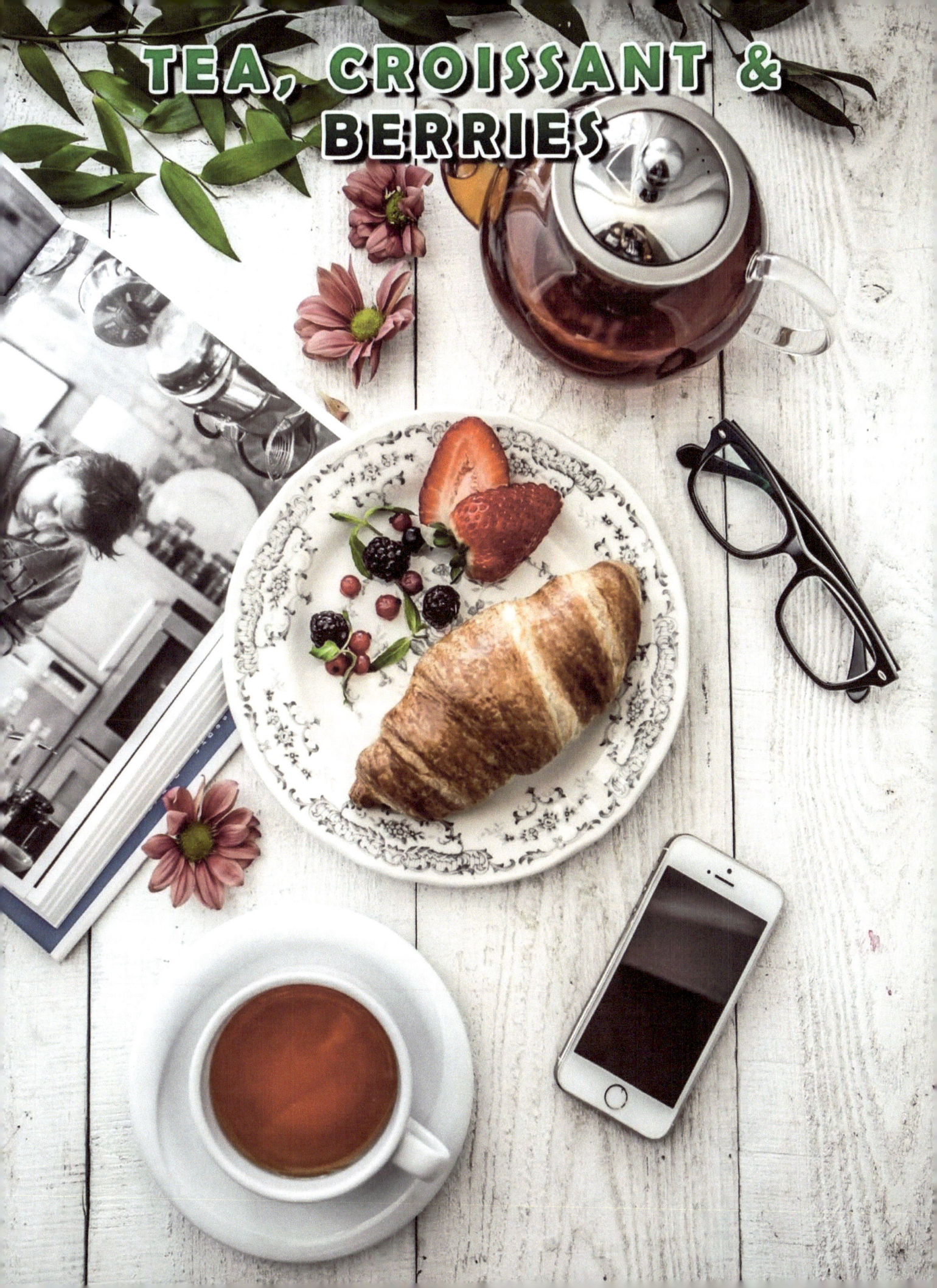

TEA, CROISSANT & BERRIES

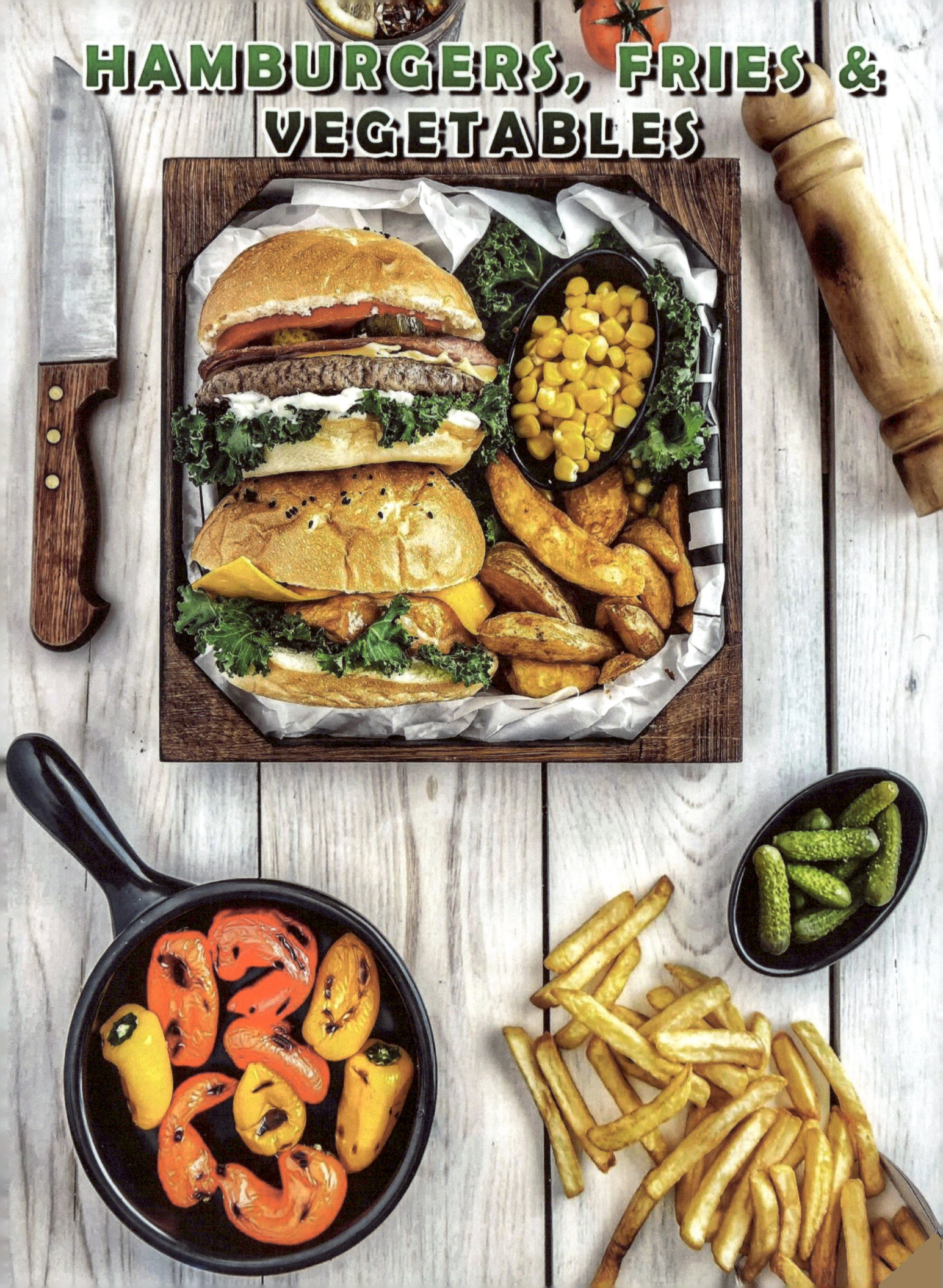

HAMBURGERS, FRIES & VEGETABLES

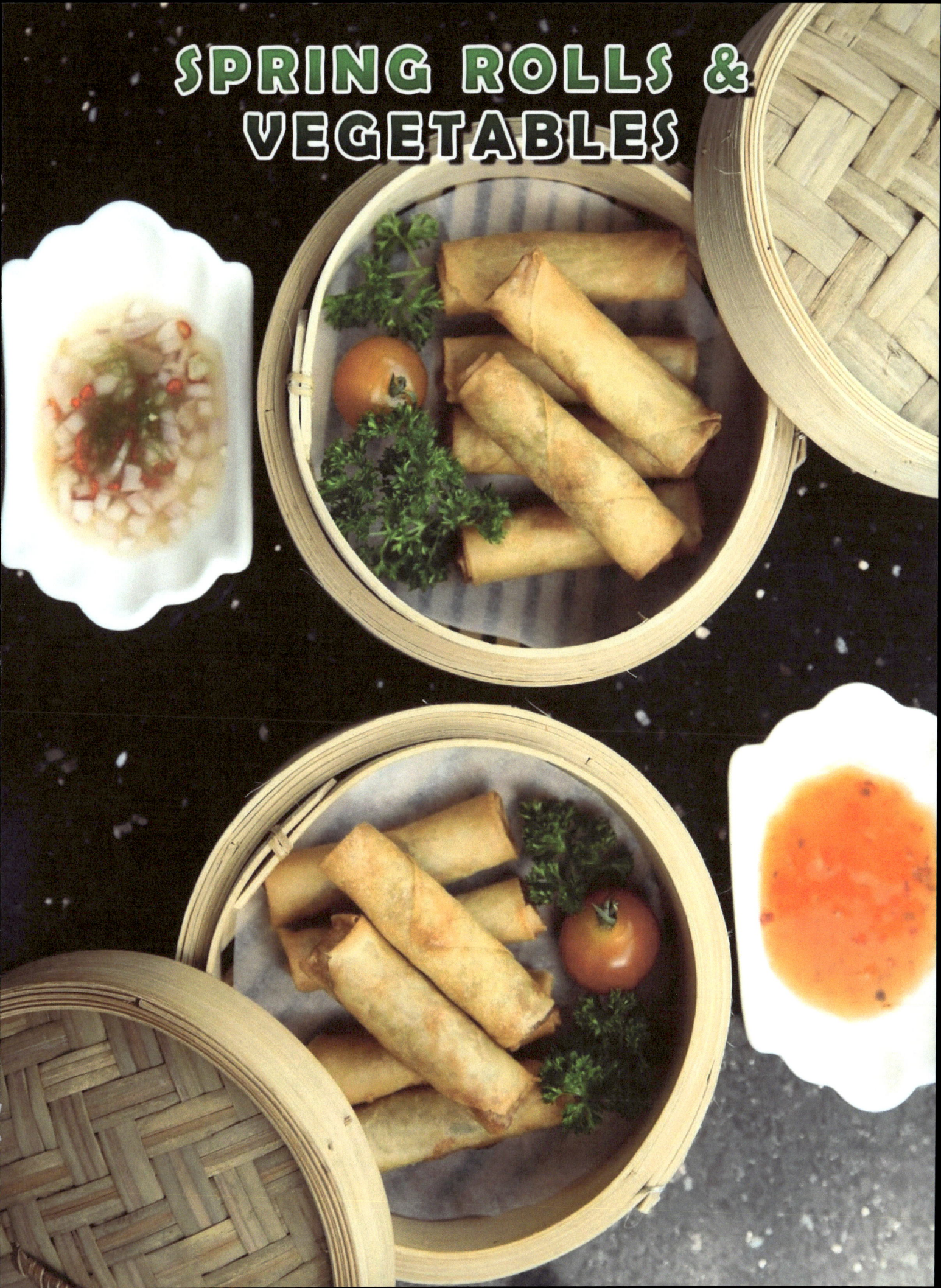

SPRING ROLLS & VEGETABLES

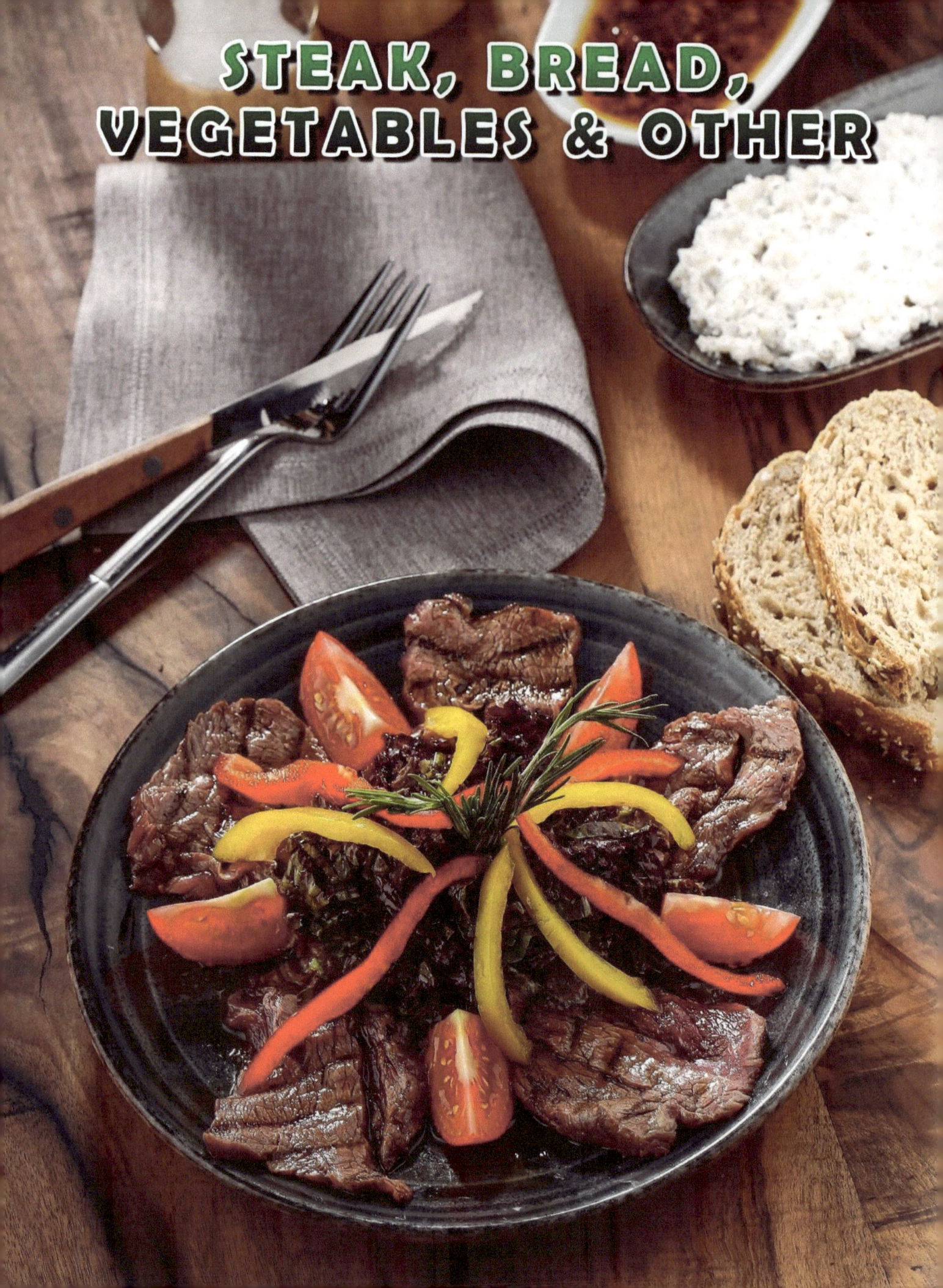

STEAK, BREAD, VEGETABLES & OTHER

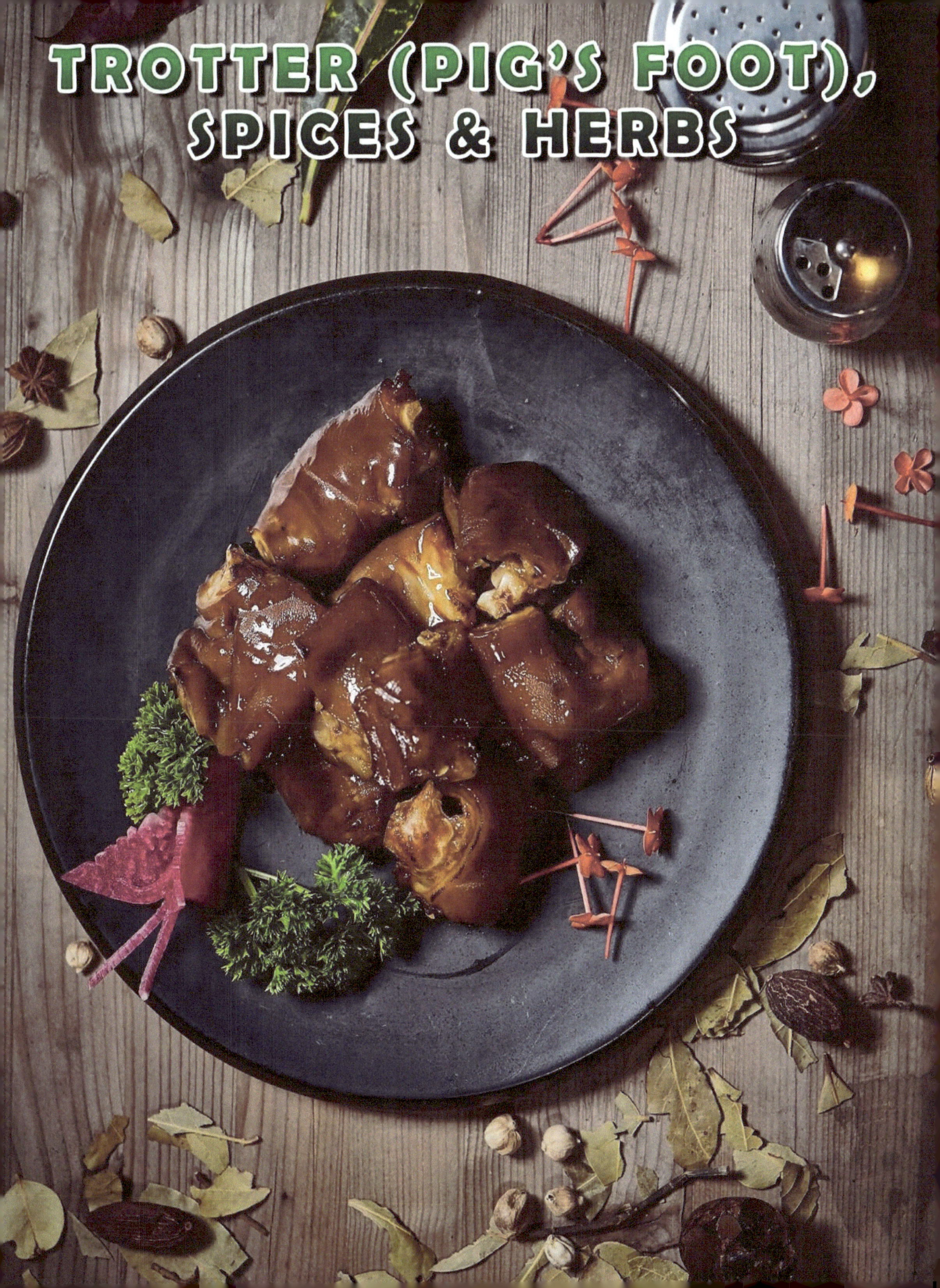

TROTTER (PIG'S FOOT), SPICES & HERBS

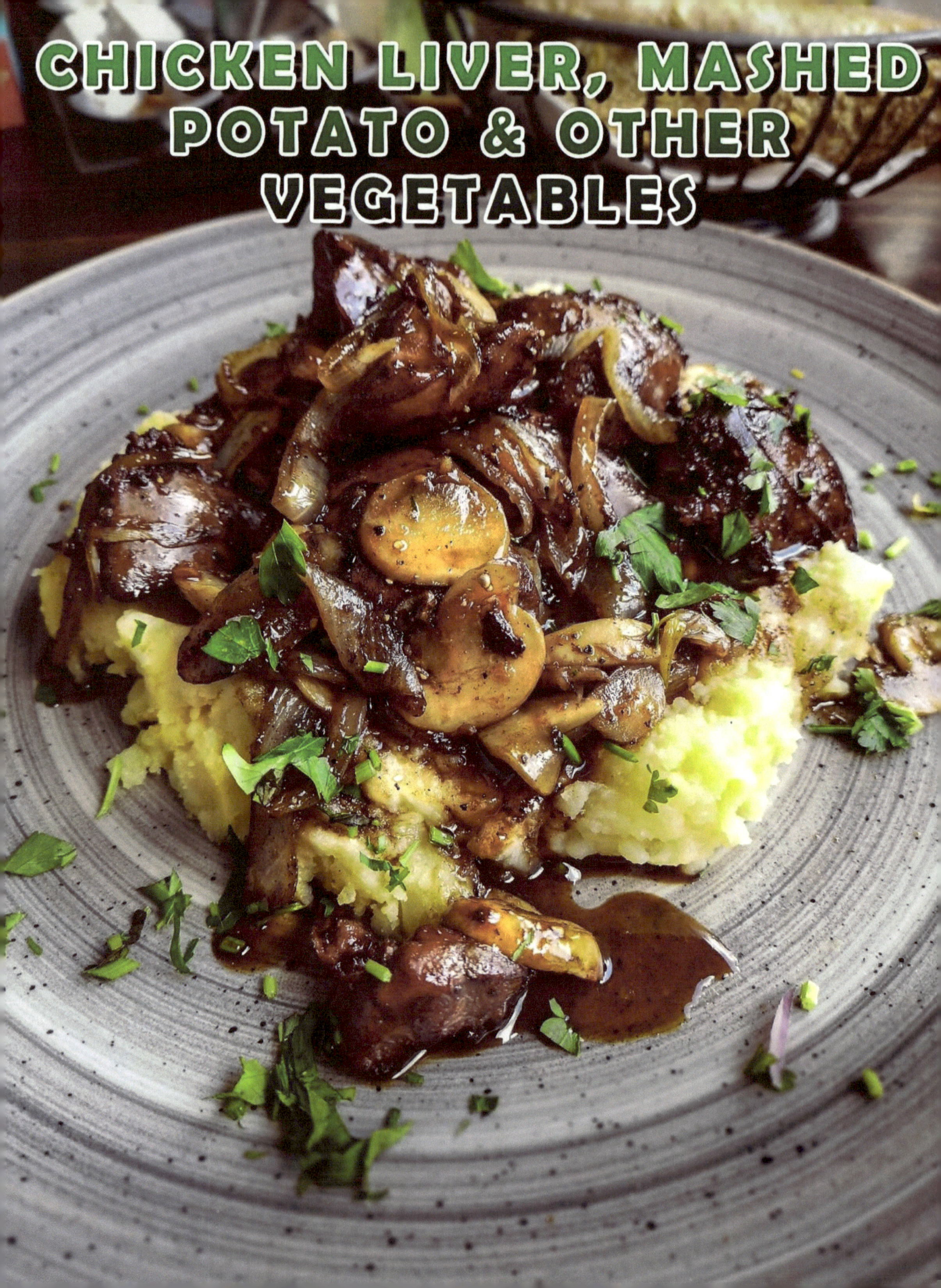

CHICKEN LIVER, MASHED POTATO & OTHER VEGETABLES

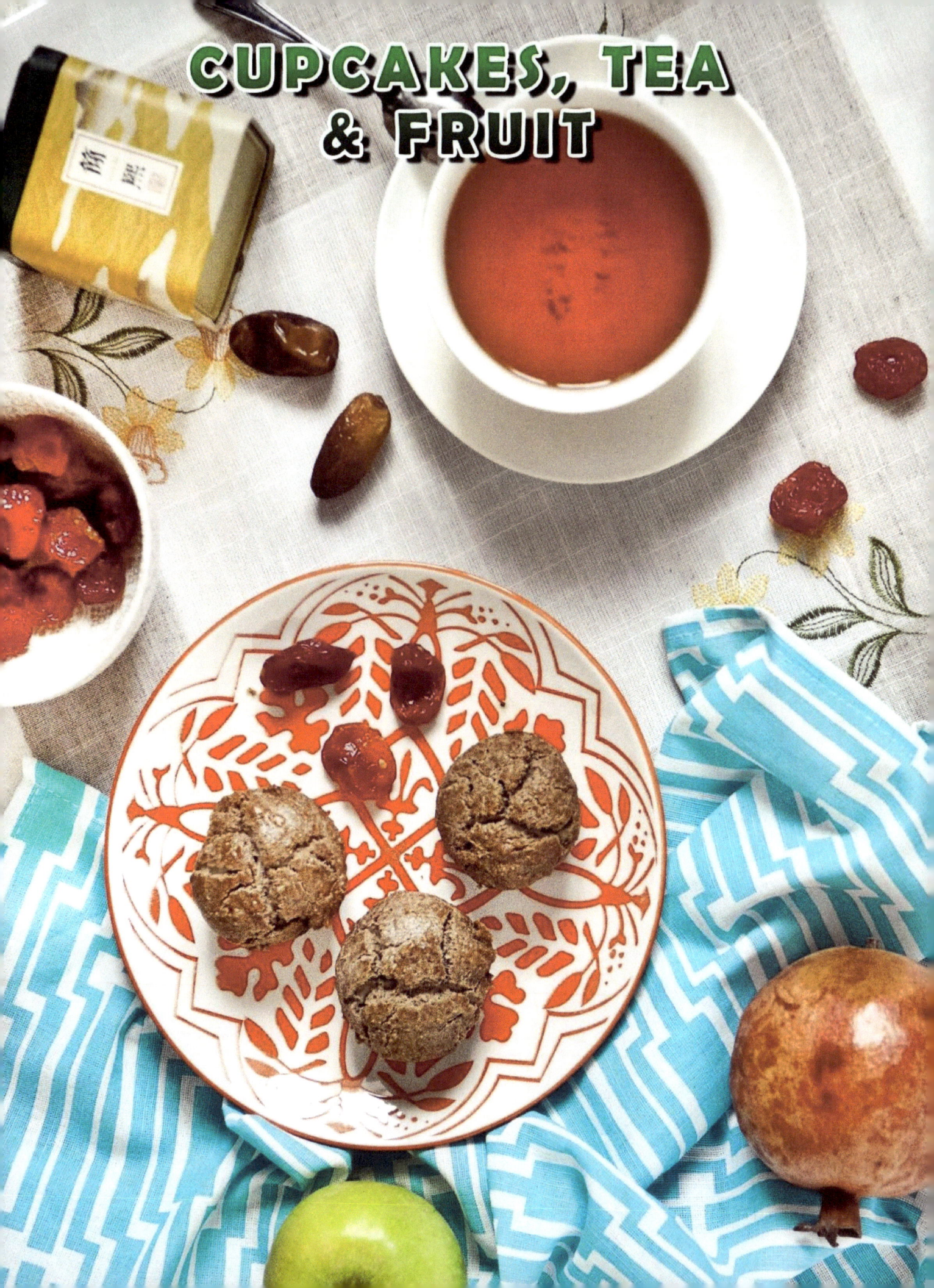

CUPCAKES, TEA & FRUIT

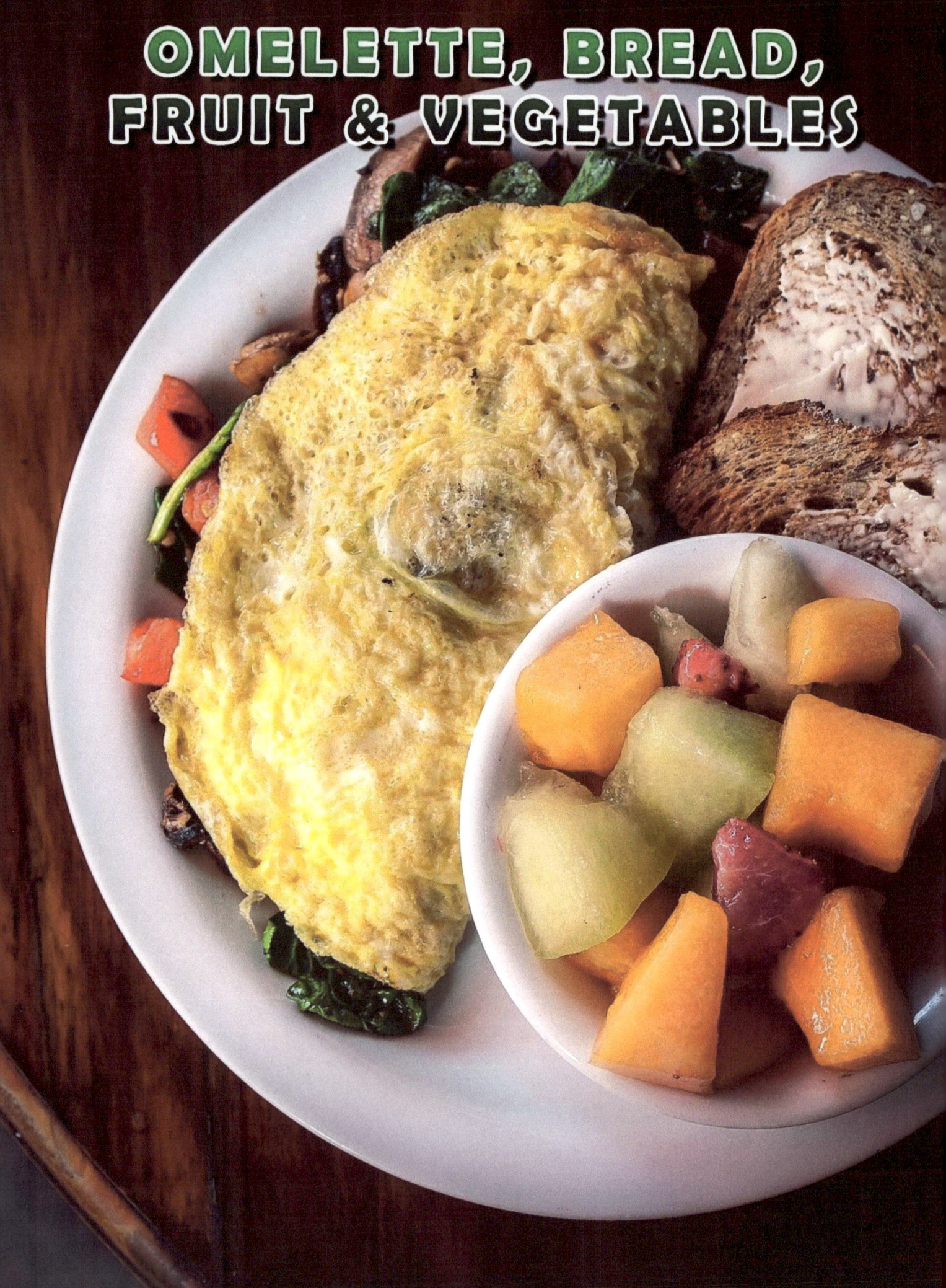

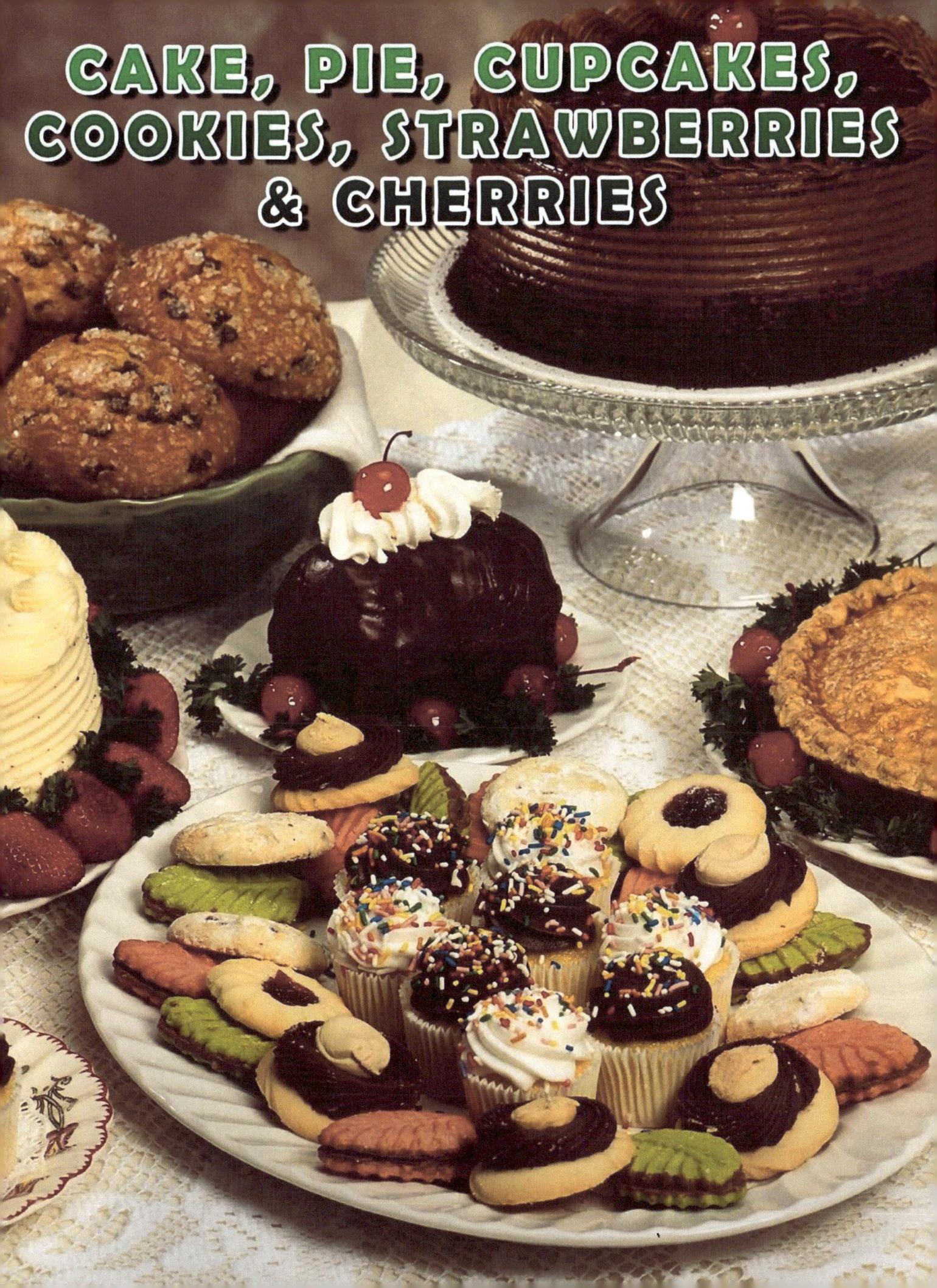

CAKE, PIE, CUPCAKES, COOKIES, STRAWBERRIES & CHERRIES

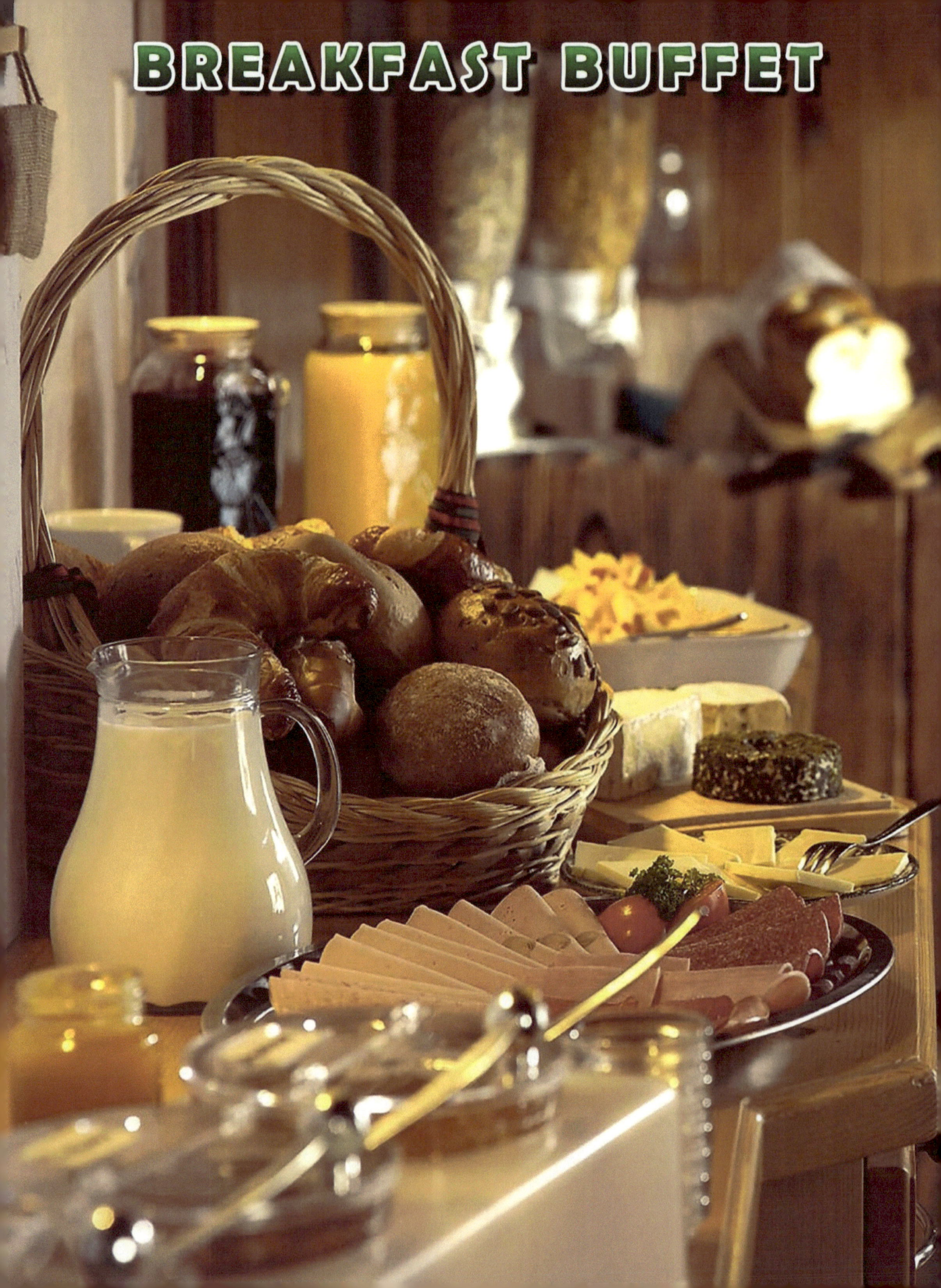

BREAKFAST BUFFET

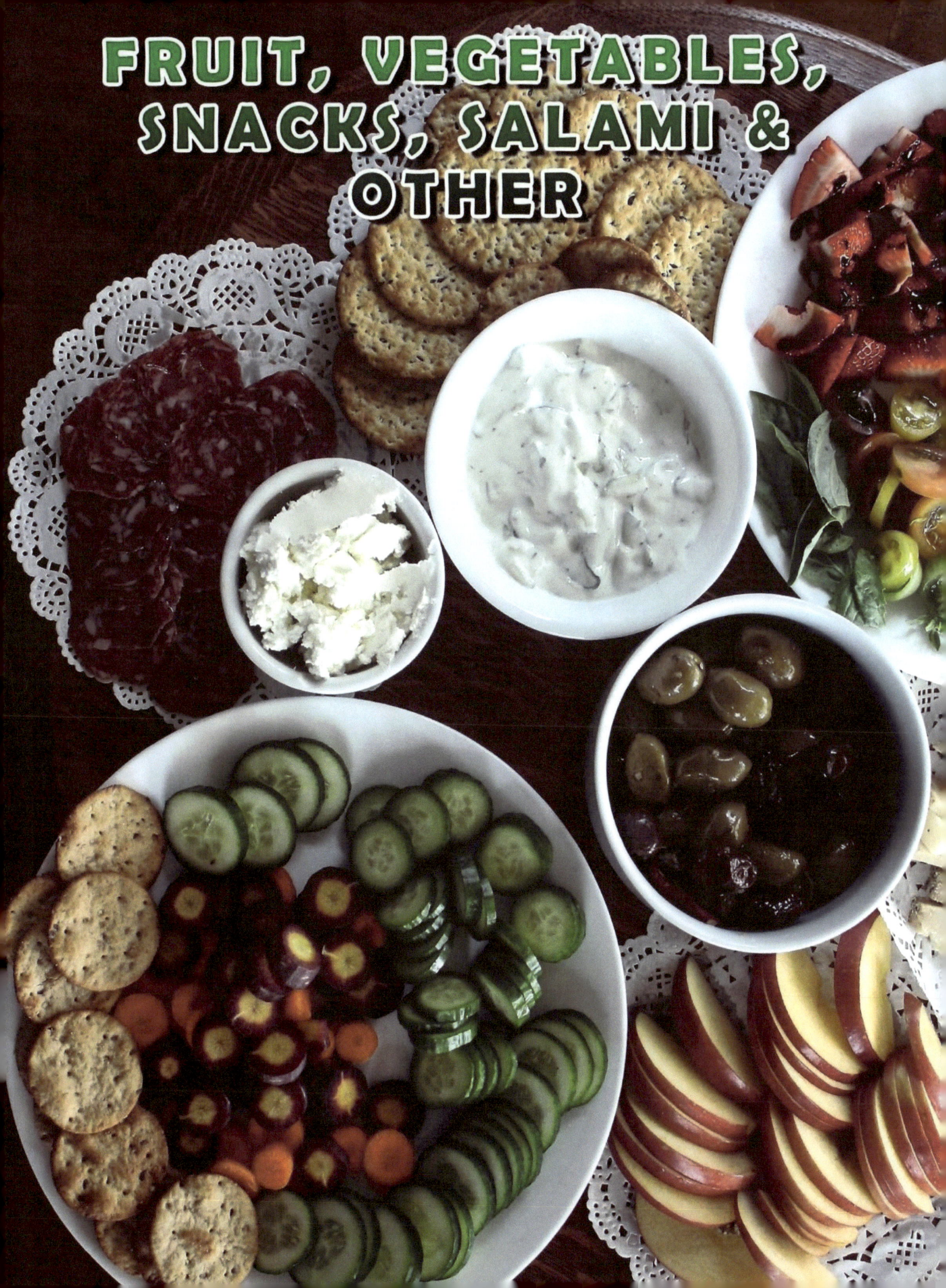

FRUIT, VEGETABLES, SNACKS, SALAMI & OTHER